Dedication

This book is dedicated to my late father, Sikuba, for teaching me how to work hard and survive; my mother, Bebi, for all the care and love she has given me; my brothers, Banana, Elias, Muloni, Lififi and the late Misheck and Stephen; sisters, Maria, Sipho, Doras and the late Simemithini; my lovely children Sobukhosi, Nqobile for tolerating my studying; Dr and Mrs Erlwanger for drastically changing the course of my life, and finally Mr Innocent Siziba, Mr Sibangiswani Jason Dube, Mr S. W. Lindow and Miss K. Fishwick for all the guidance they have given me while I have been here in England. My life has been worth it because of you, filling in at crucial times. I cherish you all.

Dr S. Ngwenya

To Veronica, Ben and Meg for their support over the years.

Mr S.W. Lindow

Acknowledgements

We should like to thank Dr David K. Gatongi MRCOG for meticulously checking the final manuscript, helping to eliminate mistakes and giving valuable suggestions. We also appreciate some good suggestions for the book from Dr Aethele Khunda MRCOG.

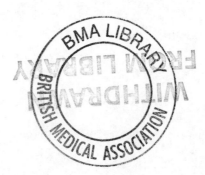

Contents

Contents

Preface

STOP! Please read this, it is very important. The examination for the MRCOG Part 2 is a truly challenging experience as the examination is very, very competitive. It is a serious examination. Obtaining the membership to the prestigious Royal College of Obstetricians and Gynaecologists (MRCOG) allows you to be internationally recognised, hence it is a well sought-after qualification. Because of its competitive nature candidates need to be well polished for this examination. From September 2006, the MRCOG Part 2 examination will have a new format, consisting of MCQs, Extended Matching Questions (EMQs) and short essays. Essays will be in two papers with a total of eight questions instead of 10 as previously. Each short answer paper will last for 1 hour 45 minutes, giving candidates only 26 minutes per essay. Short answer essays will contribute 60% of the overall mark, MCQs 25% and EMQs 15%. As you can clearly see the essays are crucial to passing or failing the examination. You need to pay particular attention to them and you need to be serious.

By the time you sit the examination, you must have gone through many essays, hence this book provides further essays to practise before the real exam. Any essay you see, take it as if you are writing the real exam. Time yourself and score your marks against those in the answers. You can only get better by polishing up. Learn the style of essay writing. Questions for the membership are mostly clinical in nature, so imagine a patient sitting in front of you. An opening sentence on the importance of the topic in Obstetrics and Gynaecology shows the examiner that you are aware of the subject. Remember to write out full sentences with paragraphs and **not** in point form. Short essays mean short essays therefore concise writing is essential. Each short essay should be one and a half sides of an A4 page. In the examination you are allowed both sides of an A4 paper and no further material is provided, even if you make a mistake. Mark allocation is meant to help you realise what is important in each topic. Each question is marked out of 20, like in the real examination.

The questions are mixed up so that you learn to tackle any question in front of you without having to condition yourself that it is an obstetrics section or gynaecology one. There are very few predictable things in life. What would you do if, owing to a clerical error, the first question in an obstetrics paper is a gynaecology one? I am sure you would answer it! Answers in this book are deliberately given in short form to help you remember and retain this enormous amount of knowledge. This kind of form helps you to revise topics quickly, retaining only the salient points.

Finally good luck in your efforts to join this prestigious club! When you finally do join, you will see that it was worth the sweat. I hope that this book will help in your efforts.

Dr Solwayo Ngwenya, 2006

Introduction and exam tips

There will be two short answer papers, each lasting 1 hour 45 minutes with four questions in each. The questions will carry equal marks. Thus there will be approximately 26 minutes to answer each question. It is important that you do not spend too much time on one question at the expense of another.

An analysis of past papers between 1997 and 2002 (10 papers) indicates that two-thirds of the questions involved management of clinical problems or a clinical scenario, eg 'A 26-year-old woman in her first pregnancy requests a detailed scan at 18 weeks' gestation and the baby is found to have a single choroid plexus cyst. Discuss the implication of this finding and justify her management.' The other third are more factual, eg 'Discuss routine pregnancy dating.'

The common instructions are 'justify' (20%), 'counsel/advise' (20%), describe/summarise' (16%), 'evaluate' (12%) or 'critically analyse' (12%).

You must take into the exam two black pens (ballpoints are usually preferable to fountain pens), a ruler and an accurate watch.

Preparation

This book is not intended to teach you Obstetrics and Gynaecology but to assist you in the technique required to express your knowledge in the format necessary to pass the examination. Hard work is the key to achieve the standard required and there are no short cuts.

The exam itself will rely on the standard management applicable to British Obstetrical and Gynaecological practice. The exam will not test research knowledge or knowledge of new or untried techniques or developments. You would, however, need to be up to date with new developments provided they have found a place in current clinical practice.

Most of your preparation will come from standard texts in Obstetrics and Gynaecology, up-to-date reviews found in journals: *The Obstetrician and Gynaecologist* (RCOG publication), *The Green Top Guidelines* published by the RCOG and the journal, *Current Obstetrics and Gynaecology*.

In addition to the appropriate level of knowledge in the subject, it is necessary to practise some questions, so that flaws in technique can be improved and the ability to write concisely with acceptable handwriting is perfected.

We have seen over the years numbers of extremely good doctors who have an excellent knowledge of the subject but who fail the exam repeatedly because of the inability to conform to the timing, structure and format that the exam demands.

Technique

It is essential that you write in sentences – notes or lists are not acceptable. If there are a number of facts that need to be given, they can be given as a sentence using commas, eg 'The symptoms of endometriosis include lower abdominal pain, dyspareunia, dysmenorrhoea and infertility.' Underline the word at the start of the sentence, eg 'Endometriosis is associated with symptoms of lower abdominal pain, dyspareunia, dysmenorrhoea and infertility.' Do not underline words in the text. You must use a ruler to underline, and do not underline too many words as the emphasis will be lost.

Writing

It is essential that you write legibly. The examiner will not waste time reading a scribbled answer. What you consider to be good writing may not be easy for others to read and it is advisable that you give your practice answers to someone else to check. Remember that, with respect to handwriting, quality not quantity is important.

Timing

There are 26 minutes allocated to each question and you must not go over time. If your answer is well structured and planned you will be awarded the majority of marks before you reach the end of the question. If the answer is well structured, you have begun your answer with the most important aspects and will receive the majority of the marks. The last part of your answer may not be gaining many marks, as it is the less important aspects of the topic under discussion. It makes no sense to compromise the next answer because you have gone over time on the previous answer. The examiners will not see all of your answers together and therefore you will not be given any sympathy for running short of time and failing to complete an answer.

Reading the question

The anxiety, adrenaline and tension of the moment have led many candidates to misread the question. This is a common problem and may result in failure of an otherwise acceptable paper. You must read and then reread the question before making your answer plan, and then again after your answer plan.

Answer plan

It is essential that you do an answer plan in rough before you commence your answer. The plan should only take a few minutes to complete and, together with rereading the question, should ensure that you do not make a large omission or unusual interpretation of the question. Many candidates do not wish to 'waste time' on an answer plan, but this is a false economy, as an answer plan not only allows you to formulate your answer but also enables you to structure the answer so that you start with the most important details. You also get an idea of the scope of your answer and how much detail you need to go into, in order to finish in 26 minutes.

Structuring your answer

It is important to structure your answer, and this can be achieved by using your answer plan. Once you have a structure you can enter the details of your answer in each section of the plan. Break down your structure into examples like:

- 1st, 2nd and 3rd trimester (used in the case of 'Outline the antenatal care of a woman with cardiac disease in pregnancy')

- 1st, 2nd and 3rd stage (used in the case of 'Outline the intrapartum care of a woman with cardiac disease in pregnancy')

- History, examination and special investigations (used in 'Discuss the differential diagnosis of a woman with deep dyspareunia')

- Preoperative, intraoperative and postoperative (used in 'Discuss the ways of reducing the incidence of wound sepsis associated with an abdominal hysterectomy')

- Stage 1, stage 2, stage 3 and stage 4 (used in 'Outline the management of ovarian cancer')

- Immediate, delayed and long term (used in 'Describe the complications of radiotherapy when used to treat cervical cancer')

- Medical, laparoscopic and open surgery (used in 'Evaluate the treatment of severe endometriosis').

It is necessary to plan, breakdown and structure each question. Motto: 'Quality not quantity'.

DO

- read and then reread the question

- write a brief answer plan

- structure your answer

- underline words at the start of a paragraph

- write full sentences

- finish each question on time.

DON'T

- write in note form

- give long lists without explanation

- underline the body of text of your answer

- go overtime on any question

- scribble.

Mr Stephen Lindow, 2006

Glossary

AA	Alcoholics Anonymous
AC	abdominal circumference
ACE	angiotensin-converting enzyme
ALT	alanine aminotransferase
ARM	artificial rupture of membranes
bid	twice a day
BMI	body mass index
BP	blood pressure
BSO	bilateral salpingo-oophorectomy
C_3/C_4	complement proteins
Ca125	cancer-associated antigen for ovarian cancer
CEA	carcino-embryonic antigen
CIN	cervical intraepithelial neoplasia
CMV	cytomegalovirus
CNS	central nervous system
COCP	combined oral contraceptive pill
CRP	c-reactive protein
CT	computerised tomography
CTG	cardiotocography
CVS	chorionic villous sampling
CXR	chest-radiograph
D&C	dilatation and curettage
DHEAS	dehydroepiandosterone sulphate
DM	diabetes mellitus
DNA	deoxyribonucleic acid
DVT	deep venous thrombosis
EC	emergency contraception
ECG	electrocardiogram
ECHO	echocardiogram
ECV	external cephalic version
EFW	estimated fetal weight
eg	for example
ESR	erythrocyte sedimentation rate
ET	endometrial thickness

EUA	examination under anaesthesia
FBC	full blood count
FBS	fetal blood sampling
FH	fetal heart
FISH	fluorescence *in situ* hybridisation
FSE	fetal scalp electrode
FSH	follicle stimulating hormone
G&S	group and save
GA	general anaesthesia
GDM	gestational diabetes mellitus
GND	groin node dissection
GnRH-a	gonadotrophin-releasing hormone analogues/agonists
GP	general practitioner
GTN	glyceryl trinitrate
GTT	glucose tolerance test
GUM	genitourinary medicine
hCG	human chorionic gonadotrophin
HELLP syndrome	haemolysis, elevated liver enzymes, low platelets
HPV	human papillomavirus
HRT	hormone replacement therapy
ICSI	intracytoplasmic sperm injection
ICU	intensive care unit
ie	that is
IgG	immunoglobulin G
IgM	immunoglobulin M
im	intramuscularly
IOL	induction of labour
ITU	intensive therapy unit
IUCD	intrauterine contraceptive device
IUGR	intrauterine growth restriction
iv	intravenous
IVU	intravenous urogram
LA	local anaesthesia
LFTs	liver function tests
LH	luteinising hormone
LMWH	low molecular weight heparin
LSCS	lower segment caesarean section

MESA	microsurgical epididymal sperm aspiration
MRI	magnetic resonance imaging
MRSA	methicillin-resistant staphylococci
MSU	mid-stream specimen of urine
NICU	neonatal intensive care unit
NSAIDs	non-steroidal anti-inflammatory drugs
NTDs	neural tube defects
OHSS	ovarian hyperstimulation syndrome
OI	ovulation induction
PCOS	polycystic ovarian syndrome
PCR	polymerase chain reaction
PDS	polydioxanone suture
PE	pulmonary embolism
PESA	percutaneous epididymal sperm aspiration
PET	pre-eclamptic toxaemia
PGs	prostaglandins
PID	pelvic inflammatory disease
PMB	postmenopausal bleeding
PMS	premenstrual syndrome
po	per os
POD	pouch of Douglas
POF	premature ovarian failure
PPH	postpartum haemorrhage
PPROM	premature prelabour rupture of membranes
PV	per vaginam
qds	four times a day
RTA	road traffic accident
sc	subcutaneous
SCBU	special care baby unit
SGA	small for gestational age
SHBG	sex hormone binding globulin
SLE	systemic lupus erythematosus
STIs	sexually transmitted infections
T_3	triiodothyronine
T_4	thyroxine
TACE	questionnaire for assessment of alcoholism
TAH	total abdominal hysterectomy

tds	three times a day
TEDS	thromboembolic deterrent stockings
TFTs	thyroid function tests
TOF	tracheo-oesophageal fistula
TOP	termination of pregnancy
TORCH	test for toxoplasmosis, rubella, cytomegalovirus and herpes
TOT	transobturator tape
TSH	thyroid-stimulating hormone
TVS	transvaginal scan
TVT	tension-free vaginal tape
U&Es	urea and electrolytes
USI	unprotected sexual intercourse
USS	ultrasound scan
UTI	urinary tract infection
VE	vaginal examination
VTE	venous thromboembolism
VVF	vesicovaginal fistula
WCC	white cell count
WHO	World Health Organisation
WLE	wide local excision
X-match	cross match blood
XY	male genotype

Topics covered

1. Recurrent candida infection outside pregnancy
2. Echogenic bowel
3. Psychiatric illness in pregnancy
4. CMV infection in pregnancy
5. Precocious puberty
6. PPROM at 18 weeks
7. Large for dates
8. PMB
9. Alcohol abuse in pregnancy
10. HELLP syndrome
11. SLE in pregnancy
12. HPV screening
13. Azoospermia
14. Smoking in pregnancy
15. Advanced maternal age
16. Adolescent menorrhagia
17. Small for dates
18. Endometriosis
19. Consent
20. Luteal phase pregnancy
21. Hirsutism
22. Emergency contraception
23. Heart disease in pregnancy
24. Mid-trimester miscarriages
25. Dilated renal pelves
26. Toxoplasmosis infection in pregnancy
27. Polyhydramnios
28. Shoulder dystocia consequences
29. Molar pregnancy
30. Vulval cancer
31. Urinary incontinence
32. Missed miscarriage
33. Ovulation induction in PCOS
34. PID

1. Describe the management of recurrent vulvovaginal candidiasis outside of pregnancy.

....
....
....

2. A 28-year-old patient has had an anatomy scan at 20 weeks' gestation, which showed an isolated finding of echogenic bowel. How would you manage her?

....
....
....

3. A 34-year-old multiparous woman books with you at 20 weeks' gestation; she has a history of psychiatric illness in the past. Describe her further management.

....
....
....

4. A woman is 9 weeks pregnant and is suspected of being in contact with cytomegalovirus from a relative. How would you manage her?

....

....

....

5. A mother brings her 8-year-old daughter who has had a menstrual period. How would you manage the daughter?

....

....

....

6. A primiparous woman, who had amniocentesis at 18 weeks' gestation, 1 week ago, presents with ruptured membranes. How would you manage her?

....

....

....

7. A 40-year-old multiparous woman is sent to you by her midwife because of a finding of large for dates. Describe your further management.

....

....

....

8. Describe the value of investigations in a woman with postmenopausal bleeding.

....

....

....

9. At booking you learn that a woman, who is a primiparous at 14 weeks' gestation, is drinking excessive alcohol. Describe the further management of this patient.

....

....

....

10. A patient at 30 weeks' gestation is found to have confirmed HELLP syndrome. How would you manage her?

....

....

....

11. Discuss the care of a woman with systemic lupus erythematosus with antinuclear antibodies, who is 10 weeks pregnant.

....

....

....

12. What is the value of human papillomavirus testing in cervical screening?

. . . .

. . . .

. . . .

13. A married couple attends your infertility clinic and the man is found to have azoospermia. What further tests and treatments would you offer them?

. . . .

. . . .

. . . .

14. A heavy smoker books at 13 weeks' gestation. How would you manage her antenatal care?

. . . .

. . . .

. . . .

15. A 47-year-old primiparous books at 14 weeks' gestation. Discuss her antenatal, intrapartum and postnatal care.

. . . .

. . . .

. . . .

16. A 12-year-old has menorrhagia with a low haemoglobin needing hospital admission. How would you manage her?

. . . .

. . . .

. . . .

17. A 45-year-old multiparous woman is referred to you by her midwife with a history of small for dates at 34 weeks' gestation. Describe her management.

. . . .

. . . .

. . . .

18. Describe the diagnosis and treatment of endometriosis.

. . . .

. . . .

. . . .

19. What are the salient points in obtaining valid consent?

. . . .

. . . .

. . . .

20. What steps would you take to prevent pregnancy at the time of sterilisation?

. . . .

. . . .

. . . .

21. A 21-year-old complains of excessive facial hair growth. Discuss your management approach.

. . . .

. . . .

. . . .

22. A 17-year-old girl requests emergency contraception. Outline your approach to her management.

. . . .

. . . .

. . . .

23. A 28-year-old woman books with you at 12 weeks' gestation and is found to have a history of rheumatic heart disease. Describe her antenatal, labour and postnatal care.

. . . .

. . . .

. . . .

24. A 30-year-old woman with two previous mid-trimester pregnancy losses at 23 and 18 weeks books with you at 8 weeks' gestation. How would manage her?

. . . .

. . . .

. . . .

25. You see a 30-year-old patient at 20 weeks' gestation, with a scan result showing bilateral dilated renal pelves. Outline your management plan.

. . . .

. . . .

. . . .

26. A patient is 14 weeks pregnant and is suspected to have been in contact with toxoplasmosis. Discuss how you will manage her.

. . . .

. . . .

. . . .

27. A 40-year-old multiparous woman is found to have polyhydramnios at 32 weeks' gestation. Discuss your approach to her management.

. . . .

. . . .

. . . .

28. What are the risk factors for shoulder dystocia? What are the maternal, fetal and neonatal consequences of shoulder dystocia? How can it be prevented?

....

....

....

29. A 20-year-old is found to have a molar pregnancy on ultrasound scan. Outline her management.

....

....

....

30. After a vulval biopsy, a 75-year-old woman is found to have squamous cell carcinoma. Discuss her management.

....

....

....

31. How would you manage a 53-year-old woman with urinary incontinence?

....

....

....

32. After a USS, at 10 weeks' gestation, there is no fetal heart and a fetal pole of 7 mm. How will you manage the patient?

....

....

....

33. Discuss methods of ovulation induction in polycystic ovary syndrome.

....

....

....

34. A patient is admitted to the ward with a suspected acute attack of PID. How will you manage her?

....

....

....

35. Discuss the management of a breech presentation at 37 weeks' gestation.

....

....

....

36. Outline the management of a primiparous woman with an eclamptic fit at 33 weeks' gestation.

....
....
....

37. Discuss the investigations and treatments in a 43-year-old woman who has had heavy periods for 14 months.

....
....
....

38. A GP calls you to discuss a 34-weeks pregnant patient who has a herpes genitalis attack. Outline your further care.

....
....
....

39. An 18-year-old with primary amenorrhoea is found to have a blind-ending vagina. Outline your management plan.

....
....
....

40. A mother brings to you a 4-year-old girl with vaginal discharge. How will you approach this clinical problem?

. . . .

. . . .

. . . .

41. A patient with two previous preterm deliveries at 33 and 34 weeks books with you at 14 weeks' gestation. Discuss your antenatal care.

. . . .

. . . .

. . . .

42. At booking, at 12 weeks' gestation, a patient is noted to have sickle cell disease. Outline your further care.

. . . .

. . . .

. . . .

43. How will you manage a patient who has just had a vaginal delivery where the midwife thinks she has a 3rd-degree tear?

. . . .

. . . .

. . . .

44. What implications can intra-abdominal adhesions have? How can they be prevented?

. . . .

. . . .

. . . .

45. A mother brings her 17-year-old daughter, who has not had a period. Discuss your management plan of investigation.

. . . .

. . . .

. . . .

46. Describe the management of endometrial cancer.

. . . .

. . . .

. . . .

47. What are the long-term health consequences of PCOS? How can they be prevented?

. . . .

. . . .

. . . .

48. At a monochorionic twin gestation of 32 weeks, one dead twin is found. How will you manage the pregnancy?

....

....

....

49. Discuss the investigations and management in a suspected case of vesicovaginal fistula.

....

....

....

50. A 26-year-old patient, who is 26 weeks pregnant, presents with an acutely swollen left leg. Describe how you will manage her antenatal care?

....

....

....

51. A rhesus negative patient is found to have anti-D antibodies at 6 IU/ml at booking. Describe her subsequent management.

....

....

....

52. Discuss the management of a retained placenta.

....

....

....

53. A cervical biopsy has shown stage 1b squamous cell carcinoma in a 34-year-old woman. Outline your management plan.

....

....

....

54. A patient is 14 weeks pregnant and is found to have hyperthyroidism. Outline your key management plans.

....

....

....

55. Describe the complications of assisted conception management and techniques.

....

....

....

56. A 58-year-old patient has lichen sclerosus. What is your approach to her care?

. . . .

. . . .

. . . .

57. Outline the salient points in the care of twins in labour at term, where one of the twins is cephalic.

. . . .

. . . .

. . . .

58. Discuss the methods and the role of instrumental vaginal delivery in modern obstetrics.

. . . .

. . . .

. . . .

59. Outline the uses of the levonorgestrel intrauterine system (the Mirena coil).

. . . .

. . . .

. . . .

60.   Describe complications of diagnostic laparoscopy for gynaecological investigation, and how to avoid them.

. . . .

. . . .

. . . .

61.   Describe the management of an ovarian cyst, 7 cm in size, in a 27-year-old pregnant patient at 14 weeks' gestation.

. . . .

. . . .

. . . .

62.   A 26-year-old patient is referred to you who has not had a period for 9 months and has no children. Her blood tests show LH >24 IU/litre, FSH >30 IU/litre on more than two occasions. What is the diagnosis and how would you investigate and treat her?

. . . .

. . . .

. . . .

63.   A patient is 32 weeks pregnant. She is a driver in a car and is involved in a RTA. Outline your management plan.

. . . .

. . . .

. . . .

64. A patient is 16 weeks pregnant and has had diarrhoea for 2 weeks. Outline your approach to her care.

. . . .

. . . .

. . . .

65. Outline the implications of obesity in obstetrics and gynaecology.

. . . .

. . . .

. . . .

66. A 65-year-old patient is referred to you with a pelvic mass by her GP. Outline your management approach.

. . . .

. . . .

. . . .

67. A 34-year-old patient with a history of primary subfertility has had an anatomy scan at 20 weeks' gestation, and the baby is found to have a cystic hygroma. Describe her management.

. . . .

. . . .

. . . .

68. Describe the management of an ovarian cyst in a 70-year-old patient.

. . . .

. . . .

. . . .

69. A 14-weeks pregnant patient is suspected to have been in contact with parvovirus. How do you manage her?

. . . .

. . . .

. . . .

70. A 38-weeks pregnant patient is admitted with significant vaginal bleeding of 600 ml. What are the possible diagnoses and how would you manage her condition?

. . . .

. . . .

. . . .

71. A 32-weeks pregnant woman with no prior history of diabetes has had a glucose tolerance test done for persistent glucosuria; the 2-hour result is 16 mmol/litre. Outline your care plan.

. . . .

. . . .

. . . .

72. A 60-year-old patient with a history of a deep venous thrombosis consults you about taking HRT. How would you counsel her?

....

....

....

73. A woman who is 18 weeks pregnant has had an episode of vaginal bleeding 2 days ago. Her last pregnancy ended with an emergency caesarean section at 32 weeks in another country. She wants to travel to the USA by air next week. How would you counsel her?

....

....

....

74. What are the principles of palliative care in gynaecological oncology?

....

....

....

75. A 26-year-old epileptic patient who has been taking sodium valproate for 5 years comes to you for prepregnancy counselling. Outline the salient points in your consultation.

....

....

....

76. What are the complications of radiotherapy for gynaecological malignancy? How could you reduce them?

. . . .

. . . .

. . . .

77. What are the fetal and neonatal consequences of a poorly controlled pre-existing diabetes mellitus in pregnancy?

. . . .

. . . .

. . . .

78. A patient is admitted with vaginal bleeding and is suspected of having obtained an illegal abortion 2 days ago. How would you manage her?

. . . .

. . . .

. . . .

79. A 33-weeks pregnant woman is admitted with left loin pain and a fever. Outline her management.

. . . .

. . . .

. . . .

80. A woman, who is 37 weeks pregnant and who has had chicken pox recently, is referred to you with a cough and a fever. What is your approach to her care?

. . . .

. . . .

. . . .

81. Compare and contrast the tension-free vaginal tape and the transobturator tape in the treatment of urodynamic stress incontinence.

. . . .

. . . .

. . . .

82. Outline contraceptive options in a 25-year-old woman with learning difficulties.

. . . .

. . . .

. . . .

83. During an emergency caesarean section at full dilatation, there is marked uterine atony. Describe steps to manage it.

. . . .

. . . .

. . . .

84. A patient is found to be 8 weeks pregnant and has a coil *in situ*. How would you manage her?

. . . .

. . . .

. . . .

85. A patient had a caesarean section 6 days ago and comes in with an intensely painful wound and discharging pus from the wound. Describe your management plan.

. . . .

. . . .

. . . .

86. A 32-year-old nulliparous obese patient had an endometrial biopsy for persistent heavy periods and has been found to have endometrial hyperplasia. Describe your management options.

. . . .

. . . .

. . . .

87. Outline appropriate preoperative work-up for a pelvic mass where malignancy is suspected.

. . . .

. . . .

. . . .

88. Just before having an emergency caesarean section for fetal distress, the patient requests to be sterilised. She is 28 years old and has four children. How do you manage her request?

....

....

....

89. A 34-weeks pregnant woman with two previous caesarean sections requests a vaginal birth. Outline your care plan.

....

....

....

90. What is the psychosexual impact of malignancy on women's health?

....

....

....

91. Which patients need a referral to a geneticist?

....

....

....

92. What are the postnatal problems that have significant maternal morbidity and mortality?

. . . .

. . . .

. . . .

93. Outline the immediate postoperative complications following gynaecological surgery.

. . . .

. . . .

. . . .

94. A 58-year-old woman has a borderline abnormal cervical smear. Describe her management.

. . . .

. . . .

. . . .

95. What colposcopic features are used to diagnose cervical intraepithelial neoplasia?

. . . .

. . . .

. . . .

96. Discuss surgical treatment of urodynamic stress incontinence.

....

....

....

97. Compare and contrast amniocentesis and chorionic villus sampling.

....

....

....

98. Discuss peritoneal closure after an open abdominal operation.

....

....

....

99. What steps can be taken to resuscitate the distressed fetus in labour?

....

....

....

100. What are the possible causes of vulval ulcers. How would you manage them?

....

....

....

Key points are given for you to consider and/or include when answering these questions. Marks allotted to each point are indicated by numbers in brackets.

1. **Describe the management of recurrent vulvovaginal candidiasis outside of pregnancy.**

- Definition: 4 or more mycologically proven episodes in 1 year **(1)**

- It is a difficult condition to treat **(1)**

- History: previous treatments, precipitating factors such as use of antibiotics, oestrogen-containing contraception, steroids and medical condition such as diabetes mellitus **(4)**

- Examination: to check for excoriation marks on external genitalia and a characteristic vaginal discharge **(3)**

- Investigations: triple swabs which include a high vaginal swab, endocervical swab, chlamydial swab and culture for candida subtypes **(3)**

- General measures: cotton underwear, avoid douching and local irritants **(1)**

- Treatment

  - a combination of emollient creams, vaginal antifungal pessaries, oral azoles; treat other infections accordingly, eg tricomonas and chlamydia **(2)**

  - Withdraw precipitating medications and treat medical conditions **(1)**

  - Long-term suppressive treatment, eg 1 pessary/week for 6–12 months may be helpful **(2)**

  - The use of Depo provera also seems to be helpful **(1)**

  - Partner treatment seems not useful **(1)**

2. A 28-year-old patient has had an anatomy scan at 20 weeks'
    gestation, which showed an isolated finding of echogenic bowel.
    How would you manage her?

- Definition: bowel has echogenicity equal to or greater than fetal
  bowel with the same machine setting   (1)

- Relevance: is a soft marker for aneuploidy   (1)

- Mostly of no consequence   (1)

- Associated with Down syndrome, cystic fibrosis, CMV infection,
  swallowed blood or meconium, IUGR and stillbirth   (4)

- Counselling is needed on invasive tests, detailed anatomy scan at
  tertiary centre to rule out other defects such as heart, brain and
  kidney malformations   (3)

- Other tests to include fetal karyotype (risks explained – miscarriage
  1% with amniocentesis) and parental peripheral blood screening for
  cystic fibrosis   (4)

- Amniocentesis allows PCR check for CMV infection   (1)

- If chromosomal abnormalities, offer the option of TOP   (2)

- If normal, follow up with serial growth scans as risk of IUGR and
  stillbirth   (3)

3. **A 34-year-old multiparous woman books with you at 20 weeks' gestation; she has a history of psychiatric illness in the past. Describe her further management.**

- What was the psychiatric illness? Can be associated with maternal mortality and can recur in pregnancy or postpartum **(1)**

- Detailed history of previous episodes, severity, admissions, types/duration of treatments and current medications **(4)**

- Family history of psychiatric illness **(1)**

- Questions related to current symptoms particularly suicidal thoughts **(2)**

- Examination for general health, hygiene and self-harm **(1)**

- Address child protection issues by appropriate referral **(1)**

- Arrange psychiatric referral during the antenatal period **(4)**

- Psychiatric team to start any medication and arrange follow-up **(2)**

- Maintain postnatal vigilance – there is a risk of suicide and infanticide **(3)**

- Follow-up to involve community care givers; needed up to 3–6 months **(1)**

4. **A woman is 9 weeks pregnant and is suspected of being in contact with cytomegalovirus from a relative. How would you manage her?**

- CMV can affect the fetus in all trimesters and immunity is not lifelong **(2)**

- Small risk to fetus but potential fetal effects include chorioretinitis, deafness, microcephaly, jaundice, thrombocytopenia, hepatosplenomegaly, psychomotor retardation, IUGR and stillbirth **(6)**

- Maternal blood sample is needed to check IgM levels, repeated in 2–3 weeks; if rising, confirms maternal infection **(2)**

- If maternal infection is confirmed, fetal investigations will include amniocentesis at 16 weeks; PCR detection of CMV particles in amniotic fluid will confirm fetal infection **(2)**

- Other tests include FBS, which allows fetal CMV IgM levels to be checked **(2)**

- Detailed anatomy USS at 20 weeks to rule out structural defects **(3)**

- Antiviral agent ganciclovir does not seem to be effective in preventing fetal effects **(1)**

- If the fetus is affected, TOP may be offered **(1)**

- If declined, serial USS to identify IUGR will need special neonatal eye exam and paediatric follow-up **(1)**

5. **A mother brings her 8-year-old daughter who has had a menstrual period. How would you manage the daughter?**

- Diagnosis: precocious puberty   (1)

- Consequences: premature epiphysis closure, sexual abuse and psychological problems   (2)

- Causes: idiopathic (majority 90%), brain tumours, previous episodes of meningitis, encephalitis, McCune–Albright syndrome, ingestion of oestrogens, ovarian and adrenal oestrogen-secreting tumours   (4)

- History from mother about the possibility of some of the above causes   (1)

- Examination: height and weight measurement, general secondary sex characteristics, abdominal exam for masses and no pelvic exam   (3)

- Tests: include pelvic/renal USS, oestradiol, brain imaging skull radiograph, CT or MRI   (3)

- Consider giving GnRH agonists while investigating to prevent premature closure of epiphysis leading to short stature   (3)

- Appropriate referral if primary problem is found, eg endocrinologists   (1)

- If idiopathic causes, GnRH agonists until the age of 12   (2)

6. **A primiparous woman, who had amniocentesis at 18 weeks' gestation, 1 week ago, presents with ruptured membranes. How would you manage her?**

- Miscarriage risk with amniocentesis is 1%   (1)

- Note the exact time of rupture of membranes   (1)

- The fetus is at risk of lung hypoplasia from oligohydramnios, intrauterine infection and positional defects   (2)

- Maternal infection can be serious   (1)

- History and examination for symptoms and signs of infection such as maternal and fetal tachycardia, offensive vaginal discharge, maternal pyrexia

- Perform vaginal swabs for microscopy, culture and sensitivity   (3)

- Tests: FBC(WCC) and CRP   (1)

- Chemoprophylaxis with erythromycin 250 mg qds po reduces infective morbidity   (1)

- USS for liquor volume, fetal viability and serial growth scans 2-weekly   (3)

- Review amniocentesis results; if abnormal, offer the option of TOP   (1)

- If anhydramnios present, prognosis is poor; offer TOP   (1)

- If normal, serially monitor PV loss, maternal pulse, temperature, FBC and CRP   (3)

- If there are signs of infection, offer TOP   (1)

- If the pregnancy gets to edge of viability, give steroids and review by neonatal team   (1)

7. **A 40-year-old multiparous woman is sent to you by her midwife because of a finding of large for dates. Describe your further management.**

- History: check that gestation is correct, consider twins, previous obstetric outcomes, previous/family history of DM and exposure to infections **(4)**

- Examination: check fetal lie, position, palpate for pelvic masses and measure symphysiofundal height **(3)**

- Arrange for USS for biometric measurements and liquor volume, to rule out congenital abnormalities and uterine/ovarian masses **(2)**

- If normal fetal size and no previous poor obstetric history, return back to midwifery care **(2)**

- If polyhydraminios is detected, do a TORCH/parvovirus screen and arrange for a GTT to exclude latent DM; if GDM, refer to specialist joint diabetic clinic for diet/insulin therapy **(3)**

- If macrosomic, measure serial USS growth and liquor volume **(1)**

- Discuss timing and mode of delivery **(1)**

- Vaginal delivery is indicated if previous normal delivery particularly of large babies, but there is risk of shoulder dystocia **(1)**

- Elective LSCS is considered if previous shoulder dystocia, previous Caesareans, or non-cephalic presentation but there are maternal risks **(1)**

- IOL – no clear evidence that beneficial for macrosomia **(1)**

- Balance these risks and take in maternal wishes too **(1)**

8. **Describe the value of investigations in a woman with postmenopausal bleeding.**

- PMB is associated with endometrial hyperplasia and cancer (1)

- Most cases are due to benign causes (1)

- A TVS is an outpatient procedure: noninvasive, and also checks ovarian masses, measures ET; <5 mm the cancer risk is low; useful as a primary screening investigation to exclude endometrial cancer (3)

- Outpatient endometrial biopsy: pipelle (Vabra or Sharman), avoids inpatient procedure under GA; samples only 4% of cavity; can miss cancer; causes discomfort or slight bleeding; failure from stenosed os (6)

- Outpatient hysteroscopy: no GA, cavity seen directly, diagnoses polyps and submucosal fibroids; directed biopsies, but no D&C or polypectomy possible (4)

- Inpatient hysteroscopy: gold standard, direct panoramic view, D&C and polypectomy possible, but done under GA (3)

- Investigation should be used singly or in combination depending on the clinical circumstances (1)

- An audit of different methods can be carried out (1)

9. At booking you learn that a woman, who is a primiparous at 14 weeks' gestation, is drinking excessive alcohol. Describe the further management of this patient.

- Excessive alcohol ingestion associated with adverse fetal and maternal effects **(2)**

- Fetal effects include low birth weight, neurodevelopmental problems, fetal alcohol syndrome (dimorphic facial features, growth restriction and CNS involvement) but this is rare **(3)**

- Maternal effects include dependency and liver cirrhosis **(2)**

- History of how much alcohol is being taken and whether dependency exists using the TACE questionnaire; question about other substance abuse **(4)**

- Offer referral to cessation counsellors, AA, social services (risk of child neglect) **(3)**

- Taking >15 units/week is associated with IUGR, and >20 units/week with developmental problems **(2)**

- Do detailed USS at 18–20 weeks to rule out congenital malformations, but may not be evident on scan **(2)**

- Serial USS for growth and liquor volume **(1)**

- Offer contraception after delivery **(1)**

10. A patient at 30 weeks' gestation is found to have confirmed HELLP syndrome. How would you manage her?

- HELLP syndrome is a variant of PET, and defined as clinical picture with evidence of haemolysis, elevated liver enzymes (especially ALT) and low platelets   (1)

- Serious to the mother with a risk of fitting and cerebral haemorrhage   (1)

- Fetus is at risk of intrauterine death and iatrogenic prematurity   (1)

- Treatment is delivery, but stabilise first   (2)

- Use antihypertensives if high BP; strict fluid balance; magnesium sulphate drug of choice for seizure prophylaxis and treatment; vital signs monitoring and do serial blood tests   (5)

- Check fetal condition with a CTG, USS and biophysical profiles   (2)

- Inform on-call consultant obstetrician and anaesthetist   (1)

- Check cot in NICU, there may not be enough time to give steroids   (1)

- Once stabilised, deliver promptly, mostly likely by LSCS   (2)

- Consider intensive care and magnesium sulphate for 24 hours after delivery   (1)

- Give thromboprophylaxis until fully mobile   (1)

- HELLP syndrome can worsen after delivery, so repeat blood tests and monitor until clinical improvement, which can take up to a week   (1)

- Recurs in 17–27% of cases in future pregnancies   (1)

11. Discuss the care of a woman with systemic lupus erythematosus with antinuclear antibodies, who is 10 weeks pregnant.

- Systemic lupus erythematosus is a multisystem disorder **(2)**

- Maternal effects: PET, nephritis, arthritis and photosensitivity, VTE **(3)**

- Fetal effects: miscarriage risk high during a flare, recurrent miscarriages, preterm labour, IUGR, stillbirth and fetal heart block (if anti-Ro antibodies positive) **(2)**

- Manage jointly with physicians **(1)**

- Drugs used: avoid NSAIDs, but prednisolone, cyclosporin, azathioprine and hydroxychloroquine are safe, methotrexate is contraindicated **(2)**

- Dating scan is crucial, anatomy USS, fetal ECHO (if anti-Ro antibody positive) serial USS for growth, liquor volume and umbilical artery Doppler from 24 weeks **(3)**

- Review regularly: check BP, urine dipstick, blood tests anti-dsDNA (if rising), C_3, C_4 levels (checks disease activity if low), 24-hour protein if necessary, anti-Ro antibodies (risk of heart block, 3% if positive) **(3)**

- Treat maternal complications accordingly **(1)**

- Aim for vaginal delivery **(1)**

- Monitor for postpartum flare-up of disease **(2)**

12. **What is the value of human papillomavirus testing in cervical screening?**

- HPV is a DNA virus and is found in 99% of cervical cancer cases   **(2)**

- HPV is sexually acquired   **(2)**

- Oncogenic subtypes mostly involved are 16 and 18   **(1)**

- DNA particles can be detected by PCR   **(1)**

- Value: can triage mild dyskariotic smears to repeat in 6 months or immediate colposcopy   **(4)**

- If a smear is mildly dyskariotic and HPV negative, the risk of cancer developing is small, so a repeat smear in 6 months saves unnecessary colposcopy and treatment   **(3)**

- If a smear is mildly dyskariotic but HPV positive, the risk of cancer is high hence colposcopy is justified   **(2)**

- HPV testing can help categorise patients and return treated patients to normal recall frequency if HPV negative   **(2)**

- HPV can also be offered as a test but, because it is sexually acquired, it may be resented   **(2)**

- Many subtypes, which can increase the cost burden   **(1)**

13. A married couple attends your infertility clinic and the man is found to have azoospermia. What further tests and treatments would you offer them?

- Definition: azoospermia is confirmed by two samples with no sperm in ejaculate (2)

- Sensitive counselling and inform about need for further tests (1)

- Causes: brain tumours, testicular, chromosomal abnormalities, post-testicular problems, eg congenital bilateral absence of vas deferens, vasectomy, hernial surgery and previous epididymo-orchitis (5)

- Tests: include prolactin, FSH, LH, skull radiographs, CT, MRI, karyotype and cystic fibrosis screening (3)

- Treatment: if prolactinomas present, give bromocriptine and surgery for unshrinking tumours or if the patient is symptomatic (2)

- If patient has hypogonadotrophic hypogonadism (low FSH/LH) and fertility is desired, give gonadotrophins; alternatively, give testosterone (2)

- If chromosomal abnormalities are detected, counsel and involve geneticist (1)

- For post-testicular causes, offer reversal of previous surgery or sperm aspiration (PESA/MESA) and then do ICSI (2)

- Other options: adoption or artificial insemination by donor sperm (2)

14. **A heavy smoker books at 13 weeks' gestation. How would you manage her antenatal care?**

- Importance: smoking has increased risks of miscarriage, preterm delivery, IUGR and stillbirth secondary to abruption (3)

- Others: child neglect, sudden infant deaths, chest diseases, poor intellectual development and impaired physical growth (3)

- The mother is at risk of chest diseases, heart problems, abruption, placenta praevia and repeated bleeding (2)

- Check misuse of other substances, such as alcohol, cocaine and heroin (2)

- There is evidence that smoking is protective against pre-eclampsia (1)

- Check how much and what is being smoked (2)

- Give advice about stopping smoking; involve where necessary other people such as smoking cessation counsellors (2)

- Offer nicotine replacement therapy (2)

- Monitor for IUGR and offer serial USS for growth and liquor volume (3)

15. **A 47-year-old primiparous books at 14 weeks' gestation. Discuss her antenatal, intrapartum and postnatal care.**

- Importance: increased risk of miscarriage, chromosomal abnormalities, placenta praevia, twins, GDM, PET, IUGR and preterm   (3)

- History of pre-existing disease such as hypertension, type 2 DM and familial illnesses   (2)

- Offer dating USS; the risk of Down syndrome is high, so offer screening tests   (2)

- The age-related risk is around 1:20 so offer invasive testing; explain the risks of CVS and amniocentesis   (1)

- CVS gives quicker results but higher miscarriage rate (2%) than amniocentesis (1%)   (1)

- Detailed USS at 20 weeks   (1)

- Regular tests include BP, urine for proteins and glucosuria, and serial USS   (2)

- Do a GTT at 26 weeks   (1)

- During labour beware of dysfunctional labour and delayed 2nd stage leading to operative deliveries   (3)

- At this age there is a risk of VTE; if other factors present, consider thromboprophylaxis   (2)

- Neonatal care is important   (1)

- Offer effective contraception after delivery   (1)

16. A 12-year-old has menorrhagia with a low haemoglobin needing hospital admission. How would you manage her?

- Most likely cause is physiological   (1)

- This is a significant symptom needing investigation and treatment   (1)

- Take a full history of blood loss, painful periods and of anaemia, palpitations, tiredness, personal and family history of bleeding disorder   (4)

- Examination: general, abdominal; no pelvic examination if she is a virgin   (3)

- Tests: FBC especially platelet count, ferritin levels, clotting screen, and a USS to check for uterine and ovarian masses   (3)

- May need transfusion and haematinics according to blood indices   (1)

- If a bleeding disorder is found, refer to haematologists   (1)

- Otherwise, treatment options are mefenamic acid/tranexamic acid, COCP and progestogens (low dose not effective)   (4)

- Hysteroscopy and Mirena coil under GA in any patient refractory to medical management   (1)

- Surgery not indicated in adolescents   (1)

17. A 45-year-old multiparous woman is referred to you by her midwife with a history of small for dates at 34 weeks' gestation. Describe her management.

- Causes: wrong dates, error in examination, oligohydramnios and IUGR **(2)**

- Take previous obstetric history; check dates, current history, medical disorders, medications and recent contact with infections **(2)**

- Measure symphysiofundal height and examine the abdomen; make a clinical assessment **(1)**

- Arrange USS for biometric tests and liquor volume, using the 10th centile for AC and EFW to diagnose SGA **(2)**

- If normal USS, refer back to midwife **(1)**

- If SGA, perform umbilical artery Doppler, as evidence points to reduction in stillbirths, IOL and antenatal admissions in high-risk pregnancies **(2)**

- Do a detailed anatomy USS at 20 weeks and offer karyotyping if appropriate **(2)**

- Serially monitor 2-weekly with growth USS, liquor volume 2–3 times weekly, umbilical artery Doppler, and biophysical profiles **(3)**

- If IUGR and the umbilical artery Doppler is abnormal, absent or reversed (high risk of stillbirth), admit for twice daily CTGs; give steroids and inform NICU **(2)**

- Deliver by LSCS after considering whole clinical picture or if CTG is abnormal **(2)**

- If normally growing SGA baby, allow to deliver at term **(1)**

18. **Describe the diagnosis and treatment of endometriosis.**

- The definition of endometriosis is ectopic endometrial tissue **(1)**

- History: deep dyspareunia, dysmenorrhoea and subfertility, but others may be asymptomatic **(2)**

- Secondary symptoms include lower abdominal pain, pain on defaecation, rectal bleeding or bleeding from scars and umbilicus at time of menses **(2)**

- Examination: check for nodules in POD, fixed tender uterus and adnexal masses **(2)**

- Tests: USS (chocolate cysts), CT or MRI for rectovaginal septum deposits **(2)**

- Laparoscopy is diagnostic, with biopsies for histological confirmation of ectopic endometrial deposits, risks of GA, visceral and vascular damage **(2)**

- Establish fertility desire before treatment **(1)**

- No treatment for asymptomatic and incidental finding **(1)**

- Management: paracetamol/NSAIDs (if fertility is desired), COCP, progestogens, danazol, GnRH-a; all equally effective for pain relief **(2)**

- Mirena coil and the COCP for menorrhagia and dysmenorrhoea **(1)**

- Surgical ablation is effective in mild–moderate endometriosis and improves fertility outcomes; excision by minimal access techniques in specialised centres **(2)**

- Give information leaflets and addresses of support groups **(1)**

- There is a role for TAH and BSO plus HRT in severe cases who have completed their families **(1)**

19. What are the salient points in obtaining valid consent?

- Recognise a valid consent can be verbal or written (1)

- Valid consent has three principles: must be given by a competent patient, freely given and patient must be adequately informed (3)

- Back up with information leaflets (1)

- Must include proposed procedure, explain benefits and risks, additional procedures and those not to be done (3)

- Alternatives including the option of no treatments (2)

- Consent must be taken by the surgeon or someone familiar with the procedure and its complications (3)

- Parental consent is needed in children under the age of 16 but those deemed to be competent can give consent themselves (2)

- If the patient is not competent, use advance notice in the patient's best interest (3)

- If in conflict with family members, seek a court order (2)

20. **What steps would you take to prevent pregnancy at the time of sterilisation?**

- Luteal phase pregnancies contribute 30% of sterilisation failures **(3)**

- Failure: risk of a pregnancy either intrauterine or ectopic **(2)**

- The patient is responsible for taking effective contraception until the next period after sterilisation **(2)**

- Preoperative counselling must be documented **(1)**

- At the day of procedure, take a history of menstrual periods including last one, regularity and last episodes of sexual intercourse **(2)**

- Adequate identification of anatomy at the time of tubal occlusion **(2)**

- Perform a sensitive pregnancy test in all cases **(3)**

- If unprotected intercourse in luteal phase, offer emergency contraception if within 72 hours or reschedule operation **(3)**

- Avoid coil removal until after the next period following the procedure **(2)**

21. **A 21-year-old complains of excessive facial hair growth. Discuss your management approach.**

- Importance: can cause psychological problems and low self-esteem **(1)**

- Causes: idiopathic, PCOS, adrenal hyperplasia, ovarian and adrenal tumours and Cushings disease **(4)**

- History: family history, pattern of hair growth, onset, menses, fertility problems, acne, voice changes, baldness and clitomegaly **(3)**

- Examination: check for acne, hair growth on face, hands and legs, male pattern and sexual hair distribution **(2)**

- Tests: mid-follicular LH and FSH, TSH, DHEAS, 17-hydroxyprogesterone, SHBG, prolactin, testosterone and renal/pelvic USS **(4)**

- Medical treatment for PCOS or idiopathic causes is conservative with COCP, cyproterone acetate or Dianette (a combination of the two) **(3)**

- For adrenal hyperplasia use steroid therapy and involve endocrinologists **(2)**

- Surgery for tumours involving other specialists as necessary **(1)**

22. **A 17-year-old girl requests emergency contraception. Outline your approach to her management.**

- Importance: EC can prevent unwanted pregnancy if used up to 5 days of USI **(2)**

- History: menstrual, sexual, event of USI; check history of rape, previous contraception and other previous episodes of USI **(3)**

- Do a sensitive pregnancy test **(1)**

- Offer infection screening for STIs **(1)**

- EC of choice is levonorgestrel 0.75 mg tablets, 12 hours apart; good evidence supports taking two tablets at once; only contraindication is a pregnancy; side effects are nausea and vomiting; if tablets are taken within 24 hours they are 95% effective, 48 hours 85% effective and 72 hours 58% effective **(5)**

- Another option is a copper IUCD, which can be inserted up to 5 days of USI – 99% effective; coil risks are pelvic infection, uterine perforation and expulsion **(4)**

- The COCP is no longer used for EC and Mirena coil is not licensed as a method of EC **(2)**

- Offer safe sex advice, condoms and advise to return in 2 weeks if no period or problems occur **(1)**

- Counselling and advice on long-term contraception **(1)**

23. A 28-year-old woman books with you at 12 weeks' gestation and is found to have a history of rheumatic heart disease. Describe her antenatal, labour and postnatal care.

- Importance: heart disease contributes significantly to maternal mortality **(1)**

- History: nature and previous surgery of lesion, congenital or acquired; current medications such as warfarin for prosthetic valves; previous obstetric history; functional status; exercise tolerance and previous subacute bacterial endocarditis **(2)**

- Examine to check for heart murmurs, signs of congestive cardiac failure and subacute bacterial endocarditis **(2)**

- Counsel about maternal risks; heart failure, death, PET; fetal risks are IUGR and prematurity **(2)**

- Antenatal tests for mother to include; FBC, U&Es, ECG, CXR and ECHO **(1)**

- Fetal tests: offer serum screening, anatomy USS at 20 weeks and growth USS from 28 weeks **(2)**

- Regular joint care with cardiologists every 2 weeks; check cardiac status, BP, arrhythmias, FBC, urine dipstick and MSU **(2)**

- Antenatal anaesthetic review is needed **(1)**

- Aim for vaginal delivery; give antibiotics in labour: amoxycillin 1 g iv or vancomycin 1 g iv if allergy to penicillin, and gentamicin 120 mg iv to cover for subacute bacterial endocarditis **(1)**

- Meticulous fluid balance and offer an epidural and elective forceps delivery if heart failure occurs **(2)**

- Caesarean section for obstetric indications **(1)**

- Avoid ergometrine for 3rd stage; give oxytocin only **(1)**

- Monitor closely postnatal for 24–48 hours; give thromboprophylaxis **(1)**

- Offer contraception after delivery **(1)**

24. A 30-year-old woman with two previous mid-trimester pregnancy losses at 23 and 18 weeks books with you at 8 weeks' gestation. How would manage her?

- Importance: high risk pregnancy, possibility of cervical incompetence   (1)

- History: obstetric history, details of the losses and how they occurred, painful or painless labours, previous gynaecological history and previous cervical treatment   (2)

- Offer speculum examination to visualise the cervix and screening for bacterial vaginosis   (2)

- Treat infections accordingly   (1)

- Test for congenital or aquired thrombophillea defects   (1)

- Offer bloods and serum screening at booking, and anatomy scan at 20 weeks   (2)

- USS at booking for gestational age and signs of any uterine abnormalities   (2)

- Transvaginal USS for cervical length at 6 weeks repeated fortnightly   (2)

- If signs of cervical shortening or funnelling, offer cervical cerclage under tocolytic and antibiotic cover   (3)

- Warn about risks of infection, miscarriage and rupture of membranes resulting from cervical cerclage   (3)

- Some evidence that cervical cerclage improves pregnancy outcomes   (1)

- Remove suture at 37 weeks or if there are signs of chorioamnionitis (1)

25. **You see a 30-year-old patient at 20 weeks' gestation, with a scan result showing bilateral dilated renal pelves. Outline your management plan.**

- Importance: is a soft marker and can be associated with aneuploidy but majority are of no consequence and resolve spontaneously **(2)**

- History: past obstetric history particularly of aneuploidy, and family history of renal disease **(2)**

- Explain to couple: soft marker, need for a detailed anatomy USS to rule out other malformations or other soft markers **(4)**

- If major defects are diagnosed, counsel about TOP; if two or more soft markers present, counsel about invasive karyotyping **(2)**

- If no other defects, dilated pelves can be transient or secondary to obstructive uropathy, eg posterior urethral valves in males **(2)**

- Serial USS for growth, liquor volume and progression of dilatation **(3)**

- Alert paediatricians: baby may need antibiotics after delivery, and follow-up scans **(3)**

- May need referral to paediatric urologists if surgery is contemplated **(2)**

26. A patient is 14 weeks pregnant and is suspected to have been in contact with toxoplasmosis. Discuss how you will manage her.

- Counsel: small risk of the fetus being affected (1)

- Effects include: miscarriage, fetal hydrops, polyhydramnios, stillbirth, intracranial calcifications and neurodevelopmental problems (4)

- Toxoplasmosis is transmitted by eating food contaminated by cat and dog faeces (2)

- History: previous obstetric history, contact history and history of flu-like illnesses (3)

- Tests: toxoplasmosis IgG and IgM levels, and immunological tests for rubella, CMV and parvovirus (3)

- IgM can take up to 2–3 weeks to appear, so repeat testing is indicated (1)

- If strong suspicion of active infection, treat with spiramycin 3g/day (2)

- Detailed anatomy USS at 20 weeks (1)

- If the fetus is affected, counsel about TOP (1)

- Otherwise perform serial USS for growth and liquor volume (1)

- Does not affect future pregnancies (1)

27. A 40-year-old multiparous woman is found to have polyhydramnios at 32 weeks' gestation. Discuss your approach to her management.

- Risk of preterm rupture of membranes, preterm delivery, cord prolapse, maternal discomfort and PPH **(2)**

- Causes: idiopathic, GDM, congenital abnormalities, NTDs, bowel atresia, TOF, CNS defects, twins, hydrops and infections **(3)**

- History: previous obstetric history, GDM/DM, twin gestations, maternal flu-like illnesses and maternal discomfort **(3)**

- Examination: general, abdominal tension in uterine wall, fluid thrill, respiratory embarrassment and fetal presentation **(1)**

- Tests: TORCH/parvovirus B19 screen, detailed anatomy scan, a GTT and a USS for growth and liquor volume **(2)**

- Management depends on cause and severity **(1)**

- If GDM, refer to joint diabetic clinic for further care **(1)**

- If gross fetal abnormalities, counsel about TOP **(1)**

- If complications of twin pregnancy, refer to tertiary care **(1)**

- If no maternal symptoms on serial USS for growth and liquor volume, if maternal problems or severe polyhydramnios, consider treatment **(1)**

- Medical treatment with NSAIDs but there is a risk of premature closure of ductus arteriosus; surgical treatment with amnioreduction has a risk of ruptured membranes **(2)**

- Timing and mode of delivery: take obstetric factors into consideration – vaginal delivery has a risk of cord prolapse and abruption; if severe, an elective LSCS is reasonable **(1)**

- Involve paediatricians **(1)**

28. What are the risk factors for shoulder dystocia? What are the maternal, fetal and neonatal consequences of shoulder dystocia? How can it be prevented?

- Shoulder dystocia can have adverse maternal and fetal outcomes **(2)**

- Risk factors are previous history of shoulder dystocia, macrosomia, diabetes mellitus, postmaturity, prolonged labour and assisted vaginal delivery **(3)**

- Maternal effects are 3rd/4th degree tears, PPH and faecal incontinence **(3)**

- Fetal effects include birth asphyxia, cerebral palsy and stillbirth **(3)**

- Neonatal effects can be a fractured clavicle/humerus, Erb or Klumpke palsy **(3)**

- Prevention: hard to predict as 50% occur in normal sized babies **(1)**

- Do risk assessment at booking **(1)**

- Have trained staff at deliveries where there is high risk of shoulder dystocia **(2)**

- Risk management and training: regular 'obstetric drills' **(2)**

29. A 20-year-old is found to have a molar pregnancy on ultrasound scan. Outline her management.

- Molar pregnancy: explain the diagnosis to patient   (2)
- Tests: FBC, X-match 4 units, baseline hCG and CXR   (2)
- Obtain informed consent   (1)
- Management, suction evacuation under GA by an experienced surgeon as there are risks of perforation and bleeding   (2)
- Suction under ultrasound guidance by assistant   (1)
- Avoid PGs cervical priming and oxytocin until the uterus is evacuated   (2)
- Confirm diagnosis by histology   (1)
- Register patient with one of three trophoblastic centres in the UK; follow up by serial urine and/or blood hCG; inform her GP   (2)
- Any repeat evacuation to be discussed with the screening centre beforehand   (1)
- Chemotherapy as second-line treatment is highly successful   (1)
- Avoid pregnancy until hCG normal for 6 months; avoid the COCP until levels are normal (2)
- 99% cure rate   (1)
- Counsel patient about a low recurrence rate   (1)
- Do hCG levels 3 months after every subsequent pregnancy   (1)

30. After a vulval biopsy, a 75-year-old woman is found to have squamous cell carcinoma. Discuss her management.

- Vulval cancer is rare, prognosis depends on size and stage **(2)**
- Overall 5-year survival rate is 53% **(1)**
- Sensitive counselling **(1)**
- Tertiary cancer centre management by a multidisciplinary team **(1)**
- Tests: FBC, U&Es, LFTs, clotting screen, CXR, CT or MRI **(3)**
- For stage 1 lesions <1 cm, WLE with 1 cm margin around and beneath is done, then observation is needed **(3)**
- For stage 2 lesions >1 cm, node dissection is needed; if mid-line, bilateral GND and WLE are needed **(2)**
- If lesion is lateral, perform WLE and ipsilateral GND; may need contralateral GND if nodes are involved **(2)**
- Surgery can be disfiguring with poor wound healing and prolonged operative morbidity **(1)**
- Radiotherapy can be used before surgery or if nodal involvement present – risk of scarring and secondary malignancy **(2)**
- If adjuvant chemotherapy used, risks of systemic side effects and hair loss **(1)**
- Local recurrence can occur, hence follow up for 10 years **(1)**

31. **How would you manage a 53-year-old woman with urinary incontinence?**

- Classify the type of incontinence: detrusor overactivity, urodynamic stress incontinence and mixed type from the history and investigations **(2)**

- History: symptoms, extent on social life, leaking or urgency, previous treatments, surgery, past history of vaginal deliveries, medical illnesses (DM, neuropathies) and medications **(2)**

- Also ask about nocturia, frequency, flow and the use of pads **(1)**

- Check faecal incontinence and sexual activity **(2)**

- Examination: general, abdominal for masses, and pelvic for prolapse **(2)**

- Tests: urine dipstick, MSU, urinary diary and urodynamics **(3)**

- Treatments: conservative measures such as physiotherapy with pelvic floor exercises, weight loss, fluid restriction and bladder retraining **(2)**

- Medical treatment for detrusor overactivity, use either oxybutynin, tolterodine or trospium **(2)**

- Drugs are as effective as each other but less dry mouth occurs with trospium and tolterodine **(1)**

- For surgery for urodynamic stress incontinence, use either periurethral injections, TOT, TVT or Burch colposuspension **(2)**

- Mixed type may need a combination of treatment modalities **(1)**

32. After a USS, at 10 weeks' gestation, there is no fetal heart and a fetal pole of 7 mm. How will you manage the patient?

- Definition: missed miscarriage (2)

- In most cases, 65% are due to chromosomal abnormalities; other possible causes are idiopathic and metabolic disorders (1)

- Counsel together with partner (2)

- Brief history about previous obstetric history, medical history and drug allergies (2)

- Tests: FBC and G&S especially rhesus status (2)

- Offer options: either conservative, medical or surgical management (3)

- Advise on advantages and disadvantages of each (3)

- Patient choice is important (2)

- Send products for histology (2)

- Give leaflets, support group addresses and further counselling (1)

33. Discuss methods of ovulation induction in polycystic ovary syndrome.

- Ovulation induction can be difficult in PCOS (1)

- Counselling is essential (1)

- Clomiphene citrate 50–100 mg/day from day 2–6; side effects include nausea and vomiting, hot flushes, risk of multiple pregnancy and, rarely, ovarian hyperstimulation syndrome (3)

- Tamoxifen is similar to clomiphene and can be used too (1)

- Gonadotrophins 50–70 IU/day is effective therapy for clomiphene-resistant PCOS, higher rates of multiple pregnancy and OHSS (4)

- Laparoscopic ovarian drilling reduces LH levels; ovulation rates of 80% achieved; normalisation of LH levels leads to good pregnancy outcomes; no risk of multiple pregnancy and OHSS, but risks of GA, visceral and vascular damage, peri-ovarian adhesions and premature ovarian failure (5)

- Metformin therapy may improve menstrual regularity and spontaneous ovulation; emerging data are good; can be combined with clomiphene (3)

- Weight loss can bring about regular ovulation (2)

34. A patient is admitted to the ward with a suspected acute attack of PID. How will you manage her?

- PID has risks of chronic pelvic pain, infertility and ectopic pregnancies (2)

- History: pain onset, radiation, menses, sexual activity, contraception, past medical and surgical events (3)

- Examination: general, pulse, BP, temperature, abdominal, speculum and pelvic, to check for mucopurulent discharge and severity of excitation tenderness (2)

- Exclude surgical causes of an acute abdomen (1)

- Tests: cervical swabs for chlamydia, gonococci, anaerobes, FBC, CRP, ESR, syphilis serology, blood cultures if temperature >38 °C and a pregnancy test (4)

- Treatment: iv fluids, analgesia; one recommended regime is iv cefoxitin 2 g tds, and iv/po doxycycline 100 mg bd until patient is apyrexial, then oral doxycycline 100 mg bd plus oral metronidazole 400 mg tds for 14 days (3)

- Appraise clinical situation daily; if no response after 48–72 hours of iv antibiotics, book for a diagnostic laparoscopy, earlier if in diagnostic doubt (2)

- Review swabs; refer to GUM for contact tracing if STIs found (1)

- Remove IUCD in cases of severe PID (1)

- Counsel on prevention, consequences of PID; offer condoms and the COCP (1)

35. **Discuss the management of a breech presentation at 37 weeks' gestation.**

- Significance: associated with polyhydramnios, placenta praevia, fibroids and fetal abnormalities **(3)**

- History: previous obstetric history, maternal and fetal wellbeing **(1)**

- Examination: abdominal check for polyhydramnios, lie, position, presentation and fetal size **(1)**

- Arrange USS for fetal growth and liquor volume; check neck extension, placental site and congenital abnormalities **(2)**

- Offer ECV as it reduces breech and LSCS rates, with a 50% success rate; contraindications are IUGR, hyperextended neck, placenta praevia, PET and twins; perform near to theatre, as there is risk of fetal distress; an emergency LSCS, USS guidance and tocolysis may improve success; give anti-D if non-sensitised Rh D negative **(4)**

- With vaginal breech delivery, there is risk of head entrapment; need trained and experienced staff to do the delivery; worse perinatal outcome compared with elective LSCS in Term Breech Trial **(4)**

- Elective LSCS at 39 weeks if ECV unsuccessful or declined; chance of spontaneous turning; better perinatal outcome than vaginal breech delivery; no significant increase in adverse maternal outcomes in both groups in the Term Breech Trial **(5)**

36. **Outline the management of a primiparous woman with an eclamptic fit at 33 weeks' gestation.**

- Incidence of eclampsia in the UK is 4.9/10 000 maternities   (1)

- Secure airways and have patient lie in left lateral position   (1)

- Trigger a local protocol and call for a senior obstetrician and anaesthetist; inform paediatricians   (1)

- Get iv access with two large 14G cannulae and take bloods for FBC, U&Es, LFTs, clotting screen and G&S   (2)

- Monitor vital signs, pulse oximetry, ECG, urinary catheter (input–output chart), BP, pulse and temperature every 15 min   (2)

- Treatment: drug of choice for treatment and prophylaxis of fits is magnesium sulphate 4 g iv over 15 min, then 1 g/hour infusion; for recurrent fits, give 2 g iv over 15 minutes   (2)

- Check deep tendon reflexes as main side effect is respiratory depression; antidote for severe respiratory depression is calcium gluconate 1 g iv over 10 minutes   (1)

- If patient is still fitting, use iv diazepam 10 mg; she may need ventilation   (1)

- For high BP, use any of iv labetalol 50 mg, oral labetolol 200 mg or nifedipine 10 mg orally; alternatively use iv hydralazine 5 mg; control BP with regular medication   (3)

- Check fetal condition with a CTG; stabilise and deliver by LSCS in this case as definitive treatment   (2)

- Monitor in ITU environment for 24–48 hours and give thrombophylaxis   (2)

- Fill in an incident form   (1)

- Can recur in future pregnancies; patient may benefit from low-dose aspirin 75 mg/day from 12 weeks' gestation   (1)

37. **Discuss the investigations and treatments in a 43-year-old woman who has had heavy periods for 14 months.**

- Endometrial hyperplasia and cancer must be excluded **(2)**

- Possible causes include mostly hormonal imbalance, endometrial pathology and bleeding disorder **(2)**

- History: impact on social life, menses, cervical smear history, DM, nulliparity, family history of uterine or breast cancers and bleeding disorders **(3)**

- Examination: general wasting, supraclavicular lymphadenopathy, abdominal masses, speculum for cervical polyps and occult cervical cancer **(4)**

- Tests: FBC/ferritin levels, coagulation screen, TFTs, USS to rule out fibroids and adnexal masses, endometrial sampling or hysteroscopy and D&C **(3)**

- Treatment is according to cause; give iron therapy if patient is anaemic **(1)**

- Patient may need blood transfusion **(1)**

- If causes are idiopathic, options are: Mirena coil, mefenamic acid, tranexamic acid, cyclical progesterone, ablation, hysterectomy (especially if fibroids present); advise on advantages and disadvantages of each **(4)**

38. A GP calls you to discuss a 34-weeks pregnant patient who has a herpes genitalis attack. Outline your further care.

- Herpes genitalis may have serious perinatal morbidity and mortality **(2)**

- Fetal risks are encephalitis, pneumonitis and thrombocytopenia associated with a primary attack **(2)**

- History: onset, first or recurrent attack (but some attacks may be asymptomatic) and sexual contacts **(2)**

- Examination: check lesions and signs of bacterial infection **(2)**

- Tests: swabs for viral culture are not helpful; refer to GUM for screening of other STIs **(2)**

- Symptomatic relief for pain and treat secondary bacterial infection with antibiotics **(1)**

- May have urinary retention with catheterisation needed **(1)**

- Topical aciclovir reduces severity of attack and is safe in pregnancy **(2)**

- If first attack, risk of perinatal infection to baby is high; deliver by elective LSCS at 39 weeks **(2)**

- If recurrent attack, needs examination in labour for active lesions; if present, advise LSCS **(2)**

- If recurrent attack in labour with no lesions, aim for vaginal delivery but avoid invasive tests on baby such as FBS and FSE **(1)**

- Alert paediatricians as baby may need aciclovir post delivery **(1)**

39. An 18-year-old with primary amenorrhoea is found to have a blind-ending vagina. Outline your management plan.

- History: cyclical abdominal pains, attempts at sexual activity and family history **(3)**

- Examination: general for secondary sex characteristics; inspect vulva for a blue bulging membrane (haematocolpos) or pink membrane (transverse septum) **(3)**

- Tests: USS to check for uterus and ovaries, karyotype, FSH, LH and oestradiol **(3)**

- Management: very sensitive handling and best seen with mother **(1)**

- Offer psychological counselling **(1)**

- If haematocolpos or septum present, surgical excision is required **(1)**

- If XY karyotype, best to continue as female; perform gonadectomy as there is a risk of malignancy, and counsel about infertility and HRT **(2)**

- If vaginal atresia present, vaginal dilators can create a neovagina with 80% success rate; try first before surgery **(2)**

- Surgery involves techniques such as William's vulvovaginoplasty, Reed-McIndoe split skin graft and intestinal vaginoplasty but there are risks of scarring, malignancy and persistent purulent vaginal discharge **(3)**

- Perform regular vulvoscopy and biopsies **(1)**

40. A mother brings to you a 4-year-old girl with vaginal discharge. How will you approach this clinical problem?

- Needs sensitive handling (1)

- Possible causes: infection, intestinal worms, foreign bodies, sexual abuse, poor hygiene and, very rarely, tumours (5)

- History from mother about the possibility of sexual abuse; determine amount, colour and odour of discharge (3)

- Examine on mother's lap, with chaperone; inspect vulva, but no internal examination; check for discharge and scratch marks (3)

- Involve paediatricians (1)

- Arrange EUA; use paediatric laryngoscope to inspect inside of vagina to check the hymen; take swabs for anaerobes, gonococci, chlamydia, trichomonas; foreign bodies can be removed; take biopsies for histology (3)

- If intestinal worms are suspected, use overnight sellotape to trap them; send for microscopy (2)

- If she has been sexually abused, inform the police (1)

- Treat according to cause (1)

41. A patient with two previous preterm deliveries at 33 and 34 weeks books with you at 14 weeks' gestation. Discuss your antenatal care.

- Be aware that prematurity has an incidence of 7%, but contributes up to 75% of perinatal morbidity and mortality **(2)**

- There is a high risk (30–40% chance) of preterm delivery **(1)**

- Detailed history: obstetric, gynaecological, medical, drugs and alcohol **(3)**

- Offer booking bloods, dating and anatomy scans; take vaginal swab for bacterial vaginosis and screen for UTIs regularly **(4)**

- Role of cervical length scans and fibronectin tests is not yet clear **(1)**

- Role of cervical cerclage: may be useful to prevent preterm delivery **(1)**

- For serial growth and liquor volume scans from 28 weeks **(2)**

- If there is drug or alcohol misuse, offer specialist review and cessation programmes **(2)**

- If high index of suspicion, educate patient to come to the hospital early **(2)**

- Give steroids and tocolysis if she starts to threaten preterm labour and involve paediatricians **(2)**

42. At booking, at 12 weeks' gestation, a patient is noted to have sickle cell disease. Outline your further care.

- Fetal risks include miscarriage, preterm delivery, IUGR and stillbirth **(3)**

- It is an autosomal recessive genetic condition **(1)**

- Paternal testing is needed; if he is a carrier, there is a 50% chance of a sickler in offsprings, hence offer invasive testing, CVS or amniocentesis; if normal, all children will be carriers **(3)**

- Maternal risks include sickling crises, so regularly screen for infections, anaemia; avoid cold weather and dehydration **(3)**

- Jointly manage with haematologist; give folic acid, and give iron only if ferritin levels are low **(2)**

- Offer dating scan, anatomy scans, serial growth, liquor volume and Doppler scans from 24 weeks, 2-weekly **(1)**

- Sickling crises carry risks of arterial and venous thrombosis and bone infarcts **(2)**

- Manage with iv fluids, iv antibiotics, analgesia and thromboprophylaxis **(2)**

- Aim for vaginal delivery unless otherwise indicated **(1)**

- Deliver in a warm room; epidural is good for pain relief; avoid dehydration and continue thromboprophylaxis until fully mobile **(1)**

- Offer contraception after delivery but avoid the COCP **(1)**

43. How will you manage a patient who has just had a vaginal delivery where the midwife thinks she has a 3rd-degree tear?

- Most 3rd and 4th degree tears go undetected at delivery leading to faecal incontinence   (1)

- Approach to have a systematic examination of the perineum   (1)

- If 3rd or 4th degree tear is confirmed, inform on-call consultant, take bloods and consent, and inform anaesthetist on call   (2)

- Repair in theatre under GA or spinal block by an experienced operator; if 4th degree, consultant obstetrician or colorectal surgeon is needed   (2)

- Give intravenous broad spectrum antibiotics like co-amoxiclav while in theatre, then oral for 7 days postoperatively   (2)

- Use 3.0 PDS suture for the external sphincter repair; use end-to-end anastomosis or overlapping, as outcome is similar for both methods   (2)

- If 4th degree tear, rectal mucosa is first repaired with Vicryl 2.0   (1)

- Inform the patient of the nature of tear and possible complications, and fill in an incident form   (1)

- Postoperatively give laxatives for a week; avoid codeine-based analgesia   (2)

- Postoperatively, insert urinary catheter for 24 hours   (1)

- Give postnatal review in 6 weeks and at 3 months   (1)

- If symptomatic of faecal leakage, offer endoanal USS and manometry, and refer to colorectal surgeon for secondary repair   (2)

- Future deliveries can worsen anal incontinence; offer elective LSCS if symptomatic or has had secondary repair   (2)

44. What implications can intra-abdominal adhesions have? How can they be prevented?

- Adhesions can have significant impact on the patient, surgeon and the health service **(3)**

- Can result from previous surgery and infections **(2)**

- Can result in chronic pain, bowel obstruction, infertility, ectopic pregnancies, repeat investigations and operations **(4)**

- Reduction in the quality of life **(1)**

- Surgeon's time is taken up with repeat operations, each getting more difficult **(2)**

- The cost of bed occupancy and nursing care load is increased **(3)**

- Preventative measures: early infection treatment; good surgical techniques such as avoiding tissue desiccation, minimal use of diathermy and use of minimal access surgery **(3)**

- Use of antiadhesion solutions such as Adept provide a physical fluid barrier in peritoneal cavity and can be helpful **(2)**

45. A mother brings her 17-year-old daughter, who has not had a period. Discuss your management plan of investigation.

- Awareness that this is delayed puberty **(1)**

- Needs sensitive handling **(1)**

- Causes: constitutional, PCOS, POF, chromosomal abnormalities and outflow obstruction **(4)**

- History: other sibling, cyclical pain, hirsutism, sexual history, medical disorders, medications, previous radiotherapy, chemotherapy, weight gain or loss, age of breast and pubic hair development **(5)**

- Examination: general – height, weight, BMI, secondary sex characteristics, endocrine disease stigmata; abdominal examination for masses, and avoid an internal examination if virgin **(3)**

- Investigations: pregnancy test, pelvic USS, LH, FSH, SHBG, prolactin, oestradiol, testosterone and karyotype **(5)**

- Manage depending on the cause either conservatively, medically or surgically **(1)**

46. **Describe the management of endometrial cancer.**

- The prognosis depends on the stage and histological type   (1)

- Good prognosis for early stage or well differentiated; worst is
  serous adenocarcinoma   (2)

- Overall 5-year survival rate is 66%   (1)

- Sensitive counselling and management at tertiary cancer centre in
  multidisciplinary teams   (2)

- Baseline tests: FBC, LFTs, U&Es, clotting screen, X-match 4 units,
  CXR and MRI, preliminary stage of disease after MRI results   (3)

- Management: a radical TAH+BSO, peritoneal washings, plus
  omentectomy if aggressive types; debatable whether there is
  advantage in lymphadenectomy, hence not routinely done in UK   (3)

- Risks associated with surgery include infection, bleeding and VTE   (2)

- Final staging of disease after surgery with histology   (1)

- Adjuvant chemotherapy has no role in primary treatment and
  has risks of hair loss and secondary tumours   (2)

- Radiotherapy is used for stage 2 disease and recurrent vault
  disease   (1)

- Offer palliative care for advanced cases   (1)

- Long-term follow-up to 10 years   (1)

47. **What are the long-term health consequences of PCOS? How can they be prevented?**

- PCOS is a hormonal disorder associated with a metabolic disturbance   **(1)**

- Long-term problems arise from insulin resistance and unopposed oestrogens on the endometrium   **(2)**

- Long-term problems include DM, cardiovascular disease: hypertension and ischaemic heart disease, endometrial hyperplasia and cancer   **(4)**

- Preventative measures: good lifestyle, no smoking or alcohol, exercise (lose weight if obese)   **(3)**

- Menstrual withdrawal bleeds every 3 months; as prophylactic treatment for endometrial hyperplasia use COCP or Depo-provera injections to balance unopposed oestrogens or a Mirena coil   **(3)**

- If abnormal uterine bleeding, perform a hysteroscopy and D&C   **(2)**

- Regular blood tests: fasting glucose, GTT, triglyceride/lipid, cholesterol measurements, BP checks and fundoscopy   **(3)**

- There is a reduction in epithelial ovarian cancer   **(1)**

- Educate the patient on how to prevent complications   **(1)**

48. At a monochorionic twin gestation of 32 weeks, one dead twin is found. How will you manage the pregnancy?

- Monochorionic twins have a higher perinatal mortality than singletons **(2)**

- The remaining twin is at risk of preterm delivery, death (25%) and brain damage (25%) **(2)**

- Diagnose maternal disease, eg PET **(1)**

- Evaluate fetal wellbeing with a CTG, USS for growth, liquor volume and umbilical artery Doppler **(2)**

- The mother is at risk of coagulopathy **(1)**

- If maternal disease is present, offer steroids and deliver by LSCS if the dead twin is leading or mother wishes it **(2)**

- If no maternal disorder, delay delivery as damage has already occurred; twin–twin transfusion is an acute episode **(2)**

- Fetoscopic coagulation at tertiary level is still at a research stage **(1)**

- Do weekly platelet count and clotting screen **(1)**

- Twice weekly CTGs, umbilical artery Doppler and biophysical profiles **(2)**

- Weekly fetal brain scans to check for cystic brain lesions, 2-weekly growth and liquor volume scans **(3)**

- Offer fetocide if brain damage occurs; otherwise aim for delivery at 34 weeks **(1)**

49. **Discuss the investigations and management in a suspected case of vesicovaginal fistula.**

- Definition: a VVF is a non-anatomical channel between the bladder and vagina leading to continuous leakage of urine **(1)**

- Causes: cancer of the cervix, radiotherapy effects, surgery and obstructed labour (particularly in developing countries) **(2)**

- History: amounts of urine leaks, gynaecological surgery, obstetric, cancer and its treatment **(2)**

- Examination: general, Sims speculum and a bimanual **(2)**

- Investigations: urine dipstick, MSU, FBC, U&Es, IVU, EUA, cystoscopy, rectovaginal septum and plan the route of repair **(4)**

- Management: silicone barrier creams, treatment of infections, catheterisation for 6–8 weeks can allow spontaneous healing **(2)**

- Aim to repair after 12 weeks to allow slough to fall off, and infections and inflammation to settle down **(2)**

- Surgery; with the aid of urologists; repair via vaginal route in knee–chest position, or abdominal route **(2)**

- Postoperatively, catheterise for 14 days; check hourly drainage **(1)**

- Allow bed rest and give thromboprophylaxis **(1)**

- Repaired VVF has future delivery implications **(1)**

50. A 26-year-old patient, who is 26 weeks pregnant, presents with an acutely swollen left leg. Describe how you will manage her antenatal care?

- Diagnosis: DVT or cellulitis   (1)

- VTE contributes significantly to maternal morbidity and mortality – highest cause of maternal mortality in pregnant women in UK   (1)

- Hence any pregnant woman with signs and symptoms suggestive of VTE needs prompt therapy with anticoagulants while awaiting investigations   (1)

- A family and personal history of VTE or thrombophilia is important   (1)

- Examination: leg swelling, redness, perfusion, pulse, BP, temperature and respiratory rate   (2)

- LMWH as good as infused heparin but with less haemorrhagic side effects; give therapeutic dose (eg enoxaparin 1.5 mg/kg sc), once or twice daily; this does not cross placenta, but can cause thrombocytopenia and osteoporosis; warfarin crosses placenta and is contraindicated   (3)

- Investigations: arterial blood gases, ECG, FBC, clotting screen and Doppler scan of left leg   (2)

- If the Doppler scan is negative and clinical suspicion is low, stop LMWH   (2)

- If cellulitis present, treat with broad spectrum antibiotics   (1)

- If the Doppler scan is negative and clinical suspicion is high, continue LMWH; repeat Doppler scan in 1 week or consider a venogram   (2)

- If a DVT is confirmed, involve physicians; continue therapeutic LMWH for the rest of pregnancy and 6 weeks postnatally; serially monitor platelet count and do clotting screens   (2)

- Future implications for the next pregnancies   (2)

51. A rhesus negative patient is found to have anti-D antibodies at 6 IU/ml at booking. Describe her subsequent management.

- Isoimmunisation has occurred – there is a significant risk to the fetus **(1)**

- Risks include fetal hydrops and intrauterine death **(2)**

- Obstetric history is needed to check previous blood transfusions and sensitising events, such as surgical evacuations and pregnancies **(2)**

- Paternal blood grouping could be useful – if the father is homozygous DD, fetal effects are mostly likely to occur; if heterozygous Dd, the chance is 50% affected and 50% unaffected; if the father is rhesus negative, the fetus will also be negative **(2)**

- Serial antibody titres are needed every 2 weeks **(2)**

- Management by fetal medicine specialists **(2)**

- Detailed ultrasound scans are needed to check for fetal hydrops seen as ascites, pleural effusions and skin oedema **(2)**

- Middle cerebral artery Doppler can show blood redistribution and development of fetal anaemia **(1)**

- Serial growth scans are needed every 2 weeks **(1)**

- Invasive tests such as amniocentesis allow optical density determination of fetal haemolysis with use of Liley charts **(1)**

- If severely affected, fetal blood sampling can allow transfusions with Rh D negative blood depending on gestation **(1)**

- If viability is achieved, corticosteroids for fetal lung maturation are given and delivery done to allow *ex utero* transfusions **(2)**

- Involvement of paediatricians is essential, as neonatal jaundice may occur **(1)**

52. **Discuss the management of a retained placenta.**

- Definition: undelivered placenta after 30 minutes; it poses a
  significant risk of PPH   (2)

- Management will depend on bleeding or absence of associated
  bleeding   (1)

- If it occurs in a woman with a previous LSCS there is a risk of
  placenta accreta   (1)

- Check that the patient is stable; assess blood loss; make sure
  that the placenta is not in the vagina   (2)

- Site 2 14G cannulae; take blood for FBC; X-match 4 units   (2)

- Start an oxytocin infusion and insert a urinary catheter   (1)

- If there is significant bleeding, immediately transfer to theatre   (1)

- Arrange for manual removal in theatre if patient unstable, or if a
  trial of oxytocin infusion has failed after 30–60 minutes   (2)

- Inform the consultant on call and anaesthetist, and obtain consent
  as hysterectomy may be needed if accreta is present   (3)

- Before anaesthesia, check that the placenta has not delivered   (1)

- If not, proceed to manual removal of placenta, giving iv antibiotics
  in theatre and oral antibiotics for 5 days   (2)

- Check for vulval, vaginal, cervical and uterine trauma, and maintain
  an oxytocin infusion for 6–8 hours afterwards   (2)

53. A cervical biopsy has shown stage 1b squamous cell carcinoma in a 34-year-old woman. Outline your management plan.

- Early disease has a good prognosis with 80% survival rate at 5 years **(2)**

- Further tests include FBC, U&Es, LFTs, USS, IVU, CXR and a CT scan **(3)**

- MRI scan is better than CT as it can demonstrate depth of invasion and allow for more accurate staging **(1)**

- Clinical staging to include EUA, pelvic, parametrial and rectovaginal septum; check for tumour extension and perform a cystourethroscopy **(2)**

- Once carcinoma is clinically staged, refer to gynaecological oncologist who works in cancer centre in multidisciplinary teams **(2)**

- Discuss options of radiotherapy or surgery with patient **(1)**

- Surgery: radical hysterectomy, ie removal of a vaginal cuff, cervix, uterus and pelvic lymph nodes **(2)**

- If fertility is desired, radical trachelectomy with laparoscopic lymphadenectomy **(2)**

- Risks are ureteric, bladder and bowel damage; bleeding, thromboembolism; long-term risks include a shortened vagina and lymphocysts **(2)**

- Radiotherapy possible as first line or as adjuvant; risks of vaginal stenosis, ovarian failure and secondary malignancy **(2)**

- Long-term follow-up for 10 years **(1)**

54. A patient is 14 weeks pregnant and is found to have hyperthyroidism. Outline your key management plans.

- Untreated hyperthyroidism can have significant maternal and fetal effects (1)

- Maternal effects include high output cardiac failure, arrhythmia and thyroid storms (1)

- Fetal effects are miscarriage, prematurity, IUGR, stillbirth and fetal tachycardia (2)

- Best care given if jointly managed with endocrinologists (1)

- Possible causes are Graves disease, toxic multinodular goitre and toxic adenoma (2)

- Diagnosis: raised free T_3, free T_4, low TSH; also check thyroid autoantibodies (2)

- Treatment: short term β-blockers to prevent storms but no 'block and replace' regime (2)

- Antithyroid drugs available are carbimazole and propylthiouracil; these can cause fetal hypothroidism in high doses; side effects of carbimazole includes bone marrow suppression – patient should stop drugs and report if develops a sore throat or skin rash; both are safe in breastfeeding (5)

- Serial growth scans from 28 weeks (1)

- Surgery for suspected malignancy or pressure symptoms is best performed in mid-trimester (1)

- Radioactive iodine is contraindicated in pregnancy and breastfeeding as it causes fetal thyroid ablation and hypothyroidism (1)

- Involve paediatricians after delivery (1)

55. **Describe the complications of assisted conception management and techniques.**

- Assisted conception can cause psychological, financial and physical trauma (2)

- Drug reactions such as nausea, vomiting, skin rashes and anaphylaxis (1)

- Commonest drug used for ovulatory failure is clomiphine citrate 50–100 mg/day on days 2–6; complications include nausea, vomiting, hot flushes, multiple pregnancy and rarely OHSS; follicular tracking is needed (3)

- Fears about ovarian cancer are not proven (2)

- Gonadotrophin treatment gives higher risks of multiple pregnancy and OHSS; intense USS follicular tracking and oestradiol tests are needed (3)

- OHSS can be life threatening in its severe form, characterised by acute renal failure, fluid shifts and thrombosis (3)

- Egg retrieval has risk of bowel perforation and pelvic infection (2)

- Other complications include failed treatments, cancelled cycles, ectopic and heterotopic pregnancies (2)

- Possibility of transmitting genetic disorders, eg ICSI (2)

56. A 58-year-old patient has lichen sclerosus. What is your approach to her care?

- Inform the patient that the aetiology is unknown (1)

- It is thought to be autoimmune (2)

- It is not cancer or due to poor hygiene (3)

- Treatment involves potent corticosteroids nightly for 12 weeks, changed to less potent one which can be used sparingly according to how the patient feels (3)

- Treatment is not curative (1)

- Lifelong condition; the patient will be in charge of symptom control (2)

- Other creams, eg oestrogens, testosterone, antifungals, are not helpful (2)

- Regular long-term follow-up is needed to make sure there is no development of cancer; the risk is low at 3–5% (3)

- Vulval biopsies are needed in the presence of suspicious lesions (2)

- Involve a dermatologist in cases that are resistant to treatment (1)

57. Outline the salient points in the care of twins in labour at term, where one of the twins is cephalic.

- Twins have a higher perinatal morbidity and mortality than singletons, hence continuous electronic heart rate monitoring of both twins is mandatory   (2)

- Secure iv access with 2 large 14G cannulae; take blood for FBC and G&S   (2)

- Epidural recommended, as manipulation of second twin may be needed   (1)

- If the membranes have ruptured, site a fetal scalp electrode   (2)

- Inform paediatricians and anaesthetists   (1)

- Deliver first twin as singleton, and clamp the cord and aim to deliver the second twin within 30 minutes   (2)

- Stabilise the second twin in a longitudinal lie and monitor the FH; check for presentation by VE, USS or palpation   (2)

- Start an oxytocin infusion if there are no contractions and the FH is normal   (1)

- If the second twin is breech, perform external version   (2)

- If external version is unsuccessful, gently apply traction to the fetal legs; with contractions, deliver by assisted breech delivery   (2)

- If the FH is abnormal or transverse lie, deliver by LSCS   (2)

- Post delivery, maintain an oxytocin infusion for 6–8 hours to prevent PPH   (1)

58. **Discuss the methods and the role of instrumental vaginal delivery in modern obstetrics.**

- These are ventouse and forceps, either rotational or non-rotational   **(1)**

- Indications are maternal exhaustion, fetal distress and delay in 2nd stage   **(1)**

- Contraindications are unknown fetal position and station, inexperienced operator, one-fifth or more head palpable per abdomen   **(3)**

- Prerequisite to instrumental delivery are full cervical dilatation, head not palpable per abdomen, empty bladder, adequate analgesia, fetal position 0 or below, maternal effort possible, and contractions present   **(3)**

- First choice should be a ventouse – it causes fewer maternal injuries, requires less analgesia, but causes more fetal cephalohaematomas and retinal haemorrhages than forceps   **(3)**

- Forceps are more likely to succeed, need more analgesia but cause maternal trauma such as anal sphincter injuries, which may lead to faecal incontinence and bony fetal trauma   **(3)**

- Only one instrument should be used as more increase perinatal morbidity and mortality   **(2)**

- Pulling should continue only if there is descent of head; otherwise abandon and perform a LSCS   **(2)**

- Rotational forceps demand higher skills and must be used by those trained in their use   **(1)**

- Systematic rectal and vaginal examinations should be done at end of the procedure   **(1)**

59. Outline the uses of the levonorgestrel intrauterine system (the Mirena coil).

- Mirena coil contains levonorgestrel and releases 20 mcg/day **(2)**

- Used for contraception and is effective for 5 years **(1)**

- Low failure rate and as effective as female sterilisation **(2)**

- Not used for emergency contraception **(1)**

- Effective in menorrhagia (97% reduction in blood loss) and 30% women have no periods by 12 months **(3)**

- It has reduced hysterectomy rates **(2)**

- It can be used to control dysmenorrhoea and endometriosis **(2)**

- Reduces PID rates compared to other IUCDs **(2)**

- Can be used to treat PMS symptoms **(1)**

- Used for endometrial protection in endometrial hyperplasia **(2)**

- Used as HRT as part of a regime involving systemic oestrogens **(2)**

60. **Describe complications of diagnostic laparoscopy for gynaecological investigation, and how to avoid them.**

- Common procedure to investigate chronic pelvic pain, infertility and small adnexal masses   **(1)**

- Contraindicated in those with large pelvic masses and cardiopulmonary disease   **(2)**

- 'Blind' insertion of Veress needle and primary trocar causes risk of vascular and visceral damage   **(1)**

- High-risk patients include those with multiple previous abdominal surgery, history of endometriosis and obese patients   **(3)**

- Damage to bowel, bladder and blood vessels, and air embolism can occur   **(2)**

- Check equipment; position patient correctly and direct instruments properly   **(2)**

- Ensure a satisfactory pneumoperitoneum is produced   **(1)**

- Use guarded instruments and introduce secondary ports under direct vision   **(2)**

- Check instrument tips for bowel contents   **(1)**

- If suspected injury, leave instruments *in situ* and proceed to laparotomy, involving surgeons   **(2)**

- Use Palmer's point for entry or Hasson's method   **(2)**

- Postoperatively, observe for signs and symptoms suggestive of complications, eg tachycardia, low BP, pyrexia and increasing pain; involve surgeons if complications are suspected   **(1)**

61. **Describe the management of an ovarian cyst, 7 cm in size, in a 27-year-old pregnant patient at 14 weeks' gestation.**

- Ovarian cyst runs risks of torsion, rupture, haemorrhage, infection, causing an acute abdomen and risk of miscarriage **(3)**

- Check personal or family history of ovarian cancer, previous ovarian cysts and infertility treatments **(2)**

- Common type of cyst is a dermoid, but can be borderline or malignant, hence check for USS features, simple, complex or solid elements and ascites **(2)**

- Malignancy is rare in childbearing age group **(1)**

- Tumour markers not useful in pregnancy as they are elevated **(2)**

- Counsel patient about management conservatively with 4-weekly serial scans; the majority of cysts resolve spontaneously **(2)**

- Surgical management is appropriate if there is cyst complication or there is suspicion of malignancy **(2)**

- Risks of surgery include anaesthetic risks, bleeding, infection, miscarriage, and DVT; warn about the risk of oophorectomy **(3)**

- Check fetal wellbeing after surgery **(1)**

- Review histology results **(1)**

- If managed conservatively, book for a postnatal pelvic USS **(1)**

62. A 26-year-old patient is referred to you who has not had a period for 9 months and has no children. Her blood tests show LH >24 IU/litre, FSH >30 IU/litre on more than two occasions. What is the diagnosis and how would you investigate and treat her?

- The diagnosis is POF   (1)

- Causes are idiopathic, chromosomal, autoimmunity, metabolic, and previous treatment with radiotherapy or chemotherapy   (2)

- Check from history of siblings if they had POF, past medical and surgical history and symptoms like hot flushes and night sweats   (2)

- Inform patient sensitively of diagnosis and that she is probably infertile   (2)

- Book for chromosomal analysis and, if mosaicism with Y chromosome diagnosed, patient needs gonadectomy to prevent malignancy in testicular tissue   (2)

- Other tests include oestradiol, autoantibodies, GTT and TFTs   (2)

- Small chance of spontaneous ovarian activity leading to ovulation; hence, if pregnancy is not desired, contraception is needed   (2)

- HRT is needed for preventing osteoporosis – the combined pill can give this and be contraceptive too   (2)

- Give out information leaflets and support group addresses   (1)

- Yearly bone scans to check bone loss are recommended   (1)

- If children are desired, options are ovum donation or surrogacy (2)

- OI is not helpful   (1)

63. A patient is 32 weeks pregnant. She is a driver in a car and is involved in a RTA. Outline your management plan.

- Make rapid assessment of patient's vital signs; breathing, pulse and BP   (2)

- Give general examination to check for visible injuries and assess amount of blood loss if any, bruises and fractures   (2)

- Abdominal examination to check for distension and tenderness   (2)

- Secure iv access; send blood for FBC and G&S and Kleihauer   (3)

- May need iv fluids and blood transfusion   (1)

- If massive haemorrhage, contact on-call consultant obstetrician, anaesthetist and haematologist   (2)

- Once the mother has been stabilised, assess fetal wellbeing with a CTG   (1)

- If the patient is stable and the baby is fine, keep in for observations overnight   (1)

- Give anti-D at least 500 IU and check fetal cells with Kleihauer test if non-sensitised Rh D negative   (1)

- If there is fetal compromise, deliver by LSCS and inform paediatricians and NICU   (2)

- If there are suspected internal injuries, book for a laparotomy with involvement of surgeons, delivery by LSCS, and manage in ICU afterwards   (3)

64. A patient is 16 weeks pregnant and has had diarrhoea for 2 weeks. Outline your approach to her care.

- Get detailed history about number of motions a day, colour, odour of stools, any blood in the stool, abdominal pains, recent travel abroad, any contacts and relevant medical history such as inflammatory bowel disease   **(4)**

- Inquire if other members of the house had been similarly affected   **(1)**

- Examine patient for signs of dehydration; check BP, temperature and listen for the fetal heart   **(1)**

- Admit patient to an isolation room in the general ward or infection unit if available   **(1)**

- Take blood for FBC, CRP, U&Es, LFTs, send stool for microscopy, culture and sensitivity, parasites and ova and check ketones in the urine   **(4)**

- Give iv fluids and correct electrolyte imbalance   **(1)**

- Risk assess and give thromboprophylaxis if risk is high   **(2)**

- If there is bacterial infection, treat with antibiotics   **(1)**

- If there is no apparent cause and diarrhoea continues, involve gastroenterologists and give further management as dictated by them   **(1)**

- They will arrange for a colonoscopy to check for bowel cancer and inflammatory bowel disease, and for biopsies   **(2)**

- If inflammatory bowel disease is found, steroids can bring rapid resolution of the diarrhoea   **(2)**

65. Outline the implications of obesity in obstetrics and gynaecology.

- Gross obesity is a major risk factor for morbidity and mortality **(1)**

- Assessment of pelvic organs and obstetric assessment is difficult **(2)**

- There is increased risk of PCOS, problems with OI and lower birth rate after assisted conception **(2)**

- There is an association with endometrial cancer and postmenopausal breast cancer **(2)**

- Gross obesity is associated with PET, GDM, macrosomia, dysfunctional labour and shoulder dystocia **(2)**

- Antenatal and intrapartum fetal monitoring is a problem and can lead to poor perinatal outcomes **(2)**

- Morbidly obese patients are at a high risk of VTE **(2)**

- Anaesthetic challenges include difficulties with iv access, spinal/epidural siting and intubation **(3)**

- Surgical problems include poor pelvic access, bleeding, wound infection and dehiscence **(2)**

- Dietary modification and a suitable exercise regime are crucial **(2)**

66. A 65-year-old patient is referred to you with a pelvic mass by her GP. Outline your management approach.

- The mass could be benign or malignant hence ruling out cancer is critical   **(1)**

- Take a history of abdominal pain, discomfort, altered bowel/bladder function, gynaecological history, medical history and general health   **(3)**

- Examine for supraclavicular lymph nodes; check cachexia, palpate the liver and mass abdominally, and elicit any ascites   **(3)**

- Speculum examination to look at the cervix, do a bimanual to check the outline of the mass, its consistency, mobility and size   **(2)**

- Arrange for an urgent pelvic USS, FBC, U&Es, LFTs, and Ca125   **(3)**

- Review with results and prepare for a laparotomy to confirm diagnosis   **(2)**

- If USS findings are suspicious of cancer with ascites, solid elements or papillary projections with a raised Ca125, arrange to see patient with a relative; counsel that there is a high risk of malignancy, hence further tests are needed   **(3)**

- Arrange for a CXR and CT scan and refer to gynaecological oncologists in a cancer centre for a staging laparotomy   **(2)**

- If bowel cancer is suspected refer to surgeons   **(1)**

67. A 34-year-old patient with a history of primary subfertility has had an anatomy scan at 20 weeks' gestation, and the baby is found to have a cystic hygroma. Describe her management.

- A cystic hygroma is a swelling in the neck of the baby, a structural anomaly associated with trisomy 21 Turner's syndrome (2)

- Sensitive counselling with her partner is needed in view of the history (2)

- Prompt referral to a tertiary centre for a detailed anatomy scan to rule out other structural defects such as cardiac, renal, bowel and brain malformations (4)

- If other major defects are detected, counsel on fetocide/TOP (difficult in view of subfertility history) (3)

- If no other abnormalities, offer fetal karyotyping by performing an amniocentesis warning about 1% risk of miscarriage and ruptured membranes (3)

- If trisomy 21 is detected, offer the option of TOP (2)

- If an isolated defect, counsel over outcome, good with surgery (2)

- In future pregnancies, offer referral to tertiary unit for detailed scans and or invasive diagnostic testing (2)

68. **Describe the management of an ovarian cyst in a 70-year-old patient.**

- Postmenopausal ovarian cysts are mostly benign serous cyst
  adenomas   **(1)**

- Take a history of abdominal pain and gynaecological history,
  family history of ovarian and breast cancer   **(2)**

- Examination for general health and supraclavicular nodes, palpate
  for liver enlargement and check for ascites   **(2)**

- Arrange for a pelvic USS and tumour marker Ca125   **(2)**

- Review USS and check for the size and features of cancer such as
  ascites, solid areas, septa and papillary projections   **(2)**

- Calculate risk of malignancy index (RMI) using USS features,
  menopausal status and Ca125 levels (normal<35 IU/ml)   **(2)**

- If the RMI is low (<25), the cyst is simple, <5 cm and Ca125 level
  is normal; repeat Ca125 and USS in 3 months as 50% of cysts
  resolve; this can be done every 3 months for 1 year   **(2)**

- If it still persists, offer surgery at a gynaecology unit, taking into
  account history and patient's views   **(2)**

- If the RMI is medium, between 25–250, offer laparoscopic BSO by
  a senior gynaecologist at a cancer unit with peritoneal washings   **(2)**

- If the RMI is high (>250), refer to a cancer centre for a full staging
  laparotomy   **(2)**

- Cyst aspiration in a postmenopausal patient is not recommended   **(1)**

69. A 14-weeks pregnant patient is suspected to have been in contact with parvovirus. How do you manage her?

- Transmission is by respiratory route and vertical transmission to the baby **(2)**

- Reassure that most maternal infections do not result in fetal infection **(1)**

- History: rash, fever but may be asymptomatic **(1)**

- The fetal effects, high risk in second trimester, include non-immune hydrops fetalis, premature delivery and stillbirth **(2)**

- Maternal diagnosis to include serologically measuring parvovirus B19 and rubella antibodies, as rubella can present with the same picture **(2)**

- Parvovirus B19 IgM antibodies show recent infection; if negative but there is strong history of exposure, repeat in 2–3 weeks' time **(2)**

- If maternal infection is confirmed, perform fetal serial scans every 2 weeks for early detection of fetal hydrops; features are ascites, pleural effusions, scalp oedema and increased middle cerebral artery Doppler velocity indices **(4)**

- If fetal hydrops develops, refer to a tertiary centre for a decision on conservative care, as fetal hydrops can spontaneously resolve, or consider fetal blood sampling/intrauterine transfusion as a possibility **(3)**

- If viability is achieved, give steroids; delivery and extrauterine transfusion is an option **(2)**

- Parvovirus infection in pregnancy is not an indication for TOP **(1)**

70. A 38-weeks pregnant patient is admitted with significant vaginal bleeding of 600 ml. What are the possible diagnoses and how would you manage her condition?

- Possible diagnoses include, placenta praevia, abruption and ruptured uterus   (3)

- Prompt assessment of patient's condition is vital; summon senior help together with anaesthetic input   (2)

- Examination: determine the fetal lie, presenting part and the tone of the uterus   (2)

- Make sure that airways are secure, monitor vital signs, assess blood loss, secure two large bore iv accesses, and give crystalloids/colloids/bloods as necessary   (2)

- Send blood for X-match of at least 6 units, FBC, U&Es; clotting screen to include fibrinogen, fibrin degradation products and coagulation parameters   (2)

- USS for fetal heart and placental site   (1)

- If there is no FH and no placenta praevia, do a vaginal examination and ARM; set up an oxytocin infusion aiming for a vaginal delivery   (2)

- If placenta praevia, caesarean section is indicated   (1)

- If the FH is present and mother stabilised, deliver abdominally to empty the uterus and arrest the bleeding   (2)

- Postoperatively, monitor in ICU and give thromboprophylaxis TEDS and LMWH for 5 days or when fully mobile   (2)

- Observe for PPH and treat with an oxytocin infusion   (1)

71. A 32-weeks pregnant woman with no prior history of diabetes has had a glucose tolerance test done for persistent glucosuria; the 2-hour result is 16 mmol/litre. Outline your care plan.

- WHO definition: GDM   (2)

- History of obstetric outcomes should be taken   (1)

- Maternal complications include PET, recurrent UTIs, candida
  infections and diabetic emergencies   (2)

- Fetal complications include prematurity, macrosomia,
  polyhydramnios, stillbirth and shoulder dystocia   (2)

- Refer to a joint specialist diabetic clinic run by an obstetrician,
  physician, dietician and diabetic nurse specialists   (2)

- Initiate home glucose monitoring after appropriate diabetic advice   (1)

- Insulin regimes to start twice or three times a day; patient to keep
  a diary to help in dosages, aiming for preprandial blood glucose
  levels of 4–6 mmol/litre   (2)

- Arrange for fortnightly scans for detection of fetal macrosomia and
  polyhydramnios   (2)

- Formulate delivery plan at 36 weeks, well controlled diabetics to
  deliver at 38 weeks; if poorly controlled earlier, spontaneous
  vaginal delivery should be the aim and elective caesarean section if
  suspected macrosomia   (2)

- In labour, a glucose–potassium–insulin sliding scale should be
  given; normoglycaemia prevents neonatal hypoglycaemia; give
  continuous fetal monitoring; watch for dysfunctional labour and
  shoulder dystocia   (2)

- Post delivery, stop sliding scale, monitor glucose levels and get
  neonatal care for the baby   (1)

- For a 6 weeks' GTT, there is risk of developing type 2 DM
  (up to 60%)   (1)

72. A 60-year-old patient with a history of a deep venous thrombosis consults you about taking HRT. How would you counsel her?

- HRT is a risk factor for VTE   (2)

- Elicit from the history if the diagnosis of DVT was objectively made, and if there is any family history of VTE and thrombophilia; if unknown, test for it by a thrombophilia screen, prothrobin gene mutation and anticardiolipn antibodies   (3)

- Find out why she requires HRT   (1)

- Check risk factors for osteoporosis such as family history of osteoporosis, early menopause, steroid therapy and smoking   (2)

- Examination: look for evidence of chronic venous insufficiency, varicose veins and hypertension   (2)

- Inform that HRT is a risk factor and can cause a recurrence of VTE, hence it is not recommended especially if she has thrombophilia   (3)

- Alternatives to taking HRT include good lifestyle changes such as stopping smoking, regular exercise, taking calcium supplements and biphosphonates, β-blockers and progesterones for hot flushes   (3)

- Currently, selective oestrogen receptor modulators are considered to carry the same risk of thrombosis as oestrogen-containing HRT   (2)

- Other risks associated with HRT are breast cancer and strokes   (2)

73. A woman who is 18 weeks pregnant has had an episode of vaginal bleeding 2 days ago. Her last pregnancy ended with an emergency caesarean section at 32 weeks in another country. She wants to travel to the USA by air next week. How would you counsel her?

- Ensure that the bleeding has stopped, check placental site and fetal viability by USS and give anti-D given if patient is non-sensitised Rh D negative   (2)

- Check from history if the previous pregnancy was complicated by antepartum bleeding, PET, if the baby was small and if the baby is alive and well   (2)

- Ask about family and personal history of VTE and thrombophilia and length of the proposed flight   (2)

- Request the reason for the trip to the USA and whether she will be returning to the UK and at what gestational age? Make sure that her midwife checks her on return   (2)

- If the bleeding has settled, patient can travel but to be aware that airlines have no emergency facilities on board and that she takes appropriate medical insurance   (2)

- If she is at a low risk of VTE, advise her to restrict alcohol, tea and coffee intake, to do leg exercises, and drink plenty of water   (3)

- If she is at a high risk of VTE, offer thromboprophylaxis; TEDS, aspirin or LMWH   (2)

- Book her for anatomy scan at 20 weeks and serial growth scans from 28 weeks   (2)

- Discuss mode of delivery by 36 weeks, vaginal delivery versus repeat LSCS and risks/benefits of each   (2)

- Take maternal wishes into consideration   (1)

74. **What are the principles of palliative care in gynaecological oncology?**

- The patient must be pain free and receive sensitive care **(2)**

- Give regular pain relief rather than wait until in pain **(2)**

- Multidisciplinary team approach involves specialist pain control team, palliative care nurses, radiologists and oncologists **(3)**

- Use WHO analgesic ladder for pain relief, starting with non-opioid such as paracetamol or NSAIDs and/or adjuvants such as amitriptyline **(4)**

- If the pain persists, do not change to another drug but add an opioid, such as morphine, for mild to moderate pain to the above regime **(3)**

- If the pain becomes severe, use opioid for moderate to severe pain, such as high doses of morphine or fentanyl patches **(2)**

- Remember to give laxatives and antiemetics, treat infections and transfuse blood as is necessary **(1)**

- Keep hydrated and give adequate nutrition **(1)**

- Pain control may require radiotherapy **(1)**

- Palliative care may involve surgery to relieve obstruction to internal organs like bowel or ureters **(1)**

75. **A 26-year-old epileptic patient who has been taking sodium valproate for 5 years comes to you for prepregnancy counselling. Outline the salient points in your consultation.**

- All epileptic patients should ideally receive prepregnancy counselling (2)

- Ensure patient is on good contraception with COCP containing 50 μg oestrogen, or double doses of the mini-pill, or use Depo-provera or a coil until current issues are resolved (3)

- Give folic acid 5 mg/day for 12 weeks preconceptually to prevent NTDs, and continue during pregnancy (3)

- Jointly manage patient with neurologist, ensuring patient is fit-free and on appropriate medication (2)

- Sodium valproate is teratogenic, causing especially NTDs; changing to newer drugs like lamotrigine may be safer, monotherapy preferred (3)

- If she has been fit free for >2 years, patient can come off medication but may lose driving licence if fits recur (3)

- If fits increase, so will her medication requirements (1)

- Offer USS at 20 weeks for fetal abnormalities detection (1)

- Risk of child being epileptic is increased to 4%; if both parents are epileptic, the risk is 10% (2)

76. **What are the complications of radiotherapy for gynaecological malignancy? How could you reduce them?**

- Radiotherapy can have acute and late complications **(2)**

- Acute complications include skin reactions, cystitis, proctitis causing diarrhoea, colicky abdominal pains and organ perforation during instrumentation **(5)**

- Late complications include rectal bleeding, rectovaginal fistulae, bowel strictures leading to obstruction and perforation, severe bladder fibrosis and contractures **(5)**

- POF, vaginal stenosis and radiotherapy-induced cancer can occur **(2)**

- Pretreatment assessment helps reduce complications; check medical conditions and previous radiotherapy courses **(2)**

- Give appropriate dose of radiotherapy **(1)**

- Manage complications with analgesics, antidiarrhoeal agents and shield ovaries during treatment **(2)**

- Prescribe HRT if not contraindicated **(1)**

77. **What are the fetal and neonatal consequences of a poorly controlled pre-existing diabetes mellitus in pregnancy?**

- Poor diabetic control is associated with increased fetal morbidity and mortality (2)

- Fetal effects include miscarriage, congenital malformations, macrosomia, and growth restriction (4)

- Other effects include polyhydramnios, prematurity, stillbirth and shoulder dystocia (4)

- Neonatal effects include traumatic birth with birth asphxia, hypoglycaemia, hypocalcaemia and hypomagnesaemia (4)

- Polycythaemia, jaundice, respiratory distress and organomegaly can also occur in the neonatal period (2)

- Good glycaemic control, fetal surveillance, input from other specialists, particularly a diabetic physician, dietician and diabetic nurse specialists, can reduce these effects (2)

- Babies of DM mothers must get care in SCBU for monitoring (1)

- Prepregnancy counselling and improved glycaemic control during pregnancy can reduce these complications (1)

78. A patient is admitted with vaginal bleeding and is suspected of having obtained an illegal abortion 2 days ago. How would you manage her?

- Take a full history of last menstrual period, amount of bleeding, vaginal discharge and smell and general health of the patient **(3)**

- Check pulse, temperature, BP; give speculum and pelvic examination, obtaining a chlamydia swab, high vaginal and endocervical swabs; check the amount of bleeding, whether os is open or not, uterine size and adnexal tenderness **(3)**

- Send blood cultures, MSU, FBC, CRP and G&S **(2)**

- Set up a drip and give iv fluids and iv antibiotics that cover gram-negative and gram-positive organisms, eg a 3rd generation cephalosporin/metronidazole/doxycycline or penicillin/ aminoglycoside/metronidazole combination **(2)**

- Observe BP, pulse, oxygen saturation and urine output hourly **(1)**

- Arrange for prompt evacuation of the uterus, avoiding excessive curettage, as there is a risk of perforation and of causing Asherman syndrome **(2)**

- If there is suspected uterine perforation, a diagnostic laparoscopy and laparotomy may be needed **(2)**

- Critically ill patients have a risk of toxic shock and multiorgan failure, hence care in ICU will be needed **(3)**

- After recovery, offer contraceptive advice **(2)**

79. **A 33-weeks pregnant woman is admitted with left loin pain and a fever. Outline her management.**

- Diagnosis: most likely pyelonephritis **(1)**

- Possible complications are preterm delivery and toxic shock **(2)**

- Take a history of the type of pain, radiation, relieving factors, urinary symptoms and vomiting episodes, previous UTI or renal surgery/calculi **(2)**

- Check pulse, temperature, BP; examine abdomen for uterine contractions, renal angle tenderness, baby; do a speculum and obtain swabs, and a vaginal examination to rule out cervical dilatation **(3)**

- Do a urine dipstick, MSU, FBC, CRP, U&Es, blood cultures if temperature >38 °C and a CTG for fetal wellbeing **(4)**

- Set up iv access; give iv fluids and iv 3rd generation cephalosporin while awaiting bacteriology reports **(2)**

- If contractions start for tocolysis, give steroids and make sure cot is available or for *in utero* transfer if patient is stable **(2)**

- If patient is severely ill, repeat investigations, and consider change of antibiotics; involve microbiologist and transfer patient to ICU **(1)**

- Otherwise, continue iv antibiotics until patient is apyrexial for 24 hours, then change to oral for 7 daysl; repeat MSU in 2 weeks **(1)**

- If no response perform renal USS to exclude an obstructed kidney/perinephric abscess **(1)**

- If recurrent UTIs occur during pregnancy, opt for an IVU post delivery **(1)**

80. A woman, who is 37 weeks pregnant and who has had chicken pox recently, is referred to you with a cough and a fever. What is your approach to her care?

- Varicella pneumonia has a high maternal and fetal mortality **(2)**

- Care for her should be in an isolation ward away from antenatal patients **(3)**

- Jointly manage with chest physicians **(2)**

- On admission, take history of the cough, productive or not, and shortness of breath **(2)**

- Do a general assessment, pulse, BP, temperature, oxygen saturation; examine the chest for air entry, check for dullness and assess fetal wellbeing with a CTG **(4)**

- Investigations to include FBC, CRP, ECG, CXR, arterial blood gases and sputum for microscopy, culture and sensitivity **(3)**

- Give oxygen by face mask, iv aciclovir, and, if respiratory difficulties present, give mechanical ventilation, which improves maternal and fetal outcomes **(2)**

- If superimposed bacterial infection occurs, treat with antibiotics **(1)**

- Alert paediatricians as baby may get neonatal varicella syndrome and give varicella zoster immunoglobin and acyclovir to the neonate **(1)**

81. **Compare and contrast the tension-free vaginal tape and the transobturator tape in the treatment of urodynamic stress incontinence.**

- The TVT uses the retropubic approach, the TOT uses the transobturator route **(2)**

- Both are mid-urethral operations via a vaginal incision **(2)**

- Tape erosion can occur with both **(1)**

- Both are minimally invasive **(1)**

- Both can be done under GA or regional anaesthesia **(1)**

- TOT is a newer method while TVT has been in use for >5 years **(2)**

- TVT needs cystoscopy check, TOT does not **(2)**

- TVT is complicated by bladder perforation and retropubic bleeding **(3)**

- Both have good success rates of 60–80% cure for urodynamic stress incontinence **(2)**

- TVT has cumulative data because of its large numbers **(2)**

- TOT may replace TVT in future **(2)**

82. **Outline contraceptive options in a 25-year-old woman with learning difficulties.**

- There are explanation and consent issues and, if the patient is not able to consent, her parent/guardian or the court need to be involved **(2)**

- The COCP is an effective method but remembering to take it may be a problem, hence not a good option **(2)**

- The progesterone-only pill causes erratic bleeding and needs to be taken continuously and she may forget to take it, hence not a good option **(2)**

- Depo-provera 3-monthly injections can be a good option and can even cause amenorrhoea **(3)**

- Progesterone implants are effective for 3 years but may cause erratic bleeding and weight gain **(2)**

- An IUCD can be complicated by infection and hence not suitable, particularly if the woman has multiple partners; an intrauterine system may be appropriate and is effective for 5 years **(3)**

- Condom use is not a good option in view of her compliance but can prevent STIs **(2)**

- Female sterilisation is a permanent method, which, if requested by the patient or her guardian, must not be denied **(2)**

- Natural methods are not suitable **(2)**

83. During an emergency caesarean section at full dilatation, there is marked uterine atony. Describe steps to manage it.

- Uterine atony can cause significant maternal morbidity and mortality secondary to PPH (2)

- Promptly ask for oxytocin 5 IU iv and an infusion of 40 IU in 1 litre of saline (2)

- Compress the uterus to expel clots, and give ergometrine 0.25 mg iv (2)

- Assess blood loss if >1000 ml; inform the anaesthetist and call for senior help (2)

- Ask for blood to be X-matched, 6 units and send for a clotting screen and FBC; give crystalloids/colloids; transfuse blood if needed and involve haematologist (3)

- If catastrophic blood loss, consider transfusion of 2 units of uncross-matched blood (1)

- If the uterus remains atonic, give carboprost 0.25 mg im or intramyometrially; repeat every 15 minutes for up to 8 doses (2)

- When senior help arrives, if she is still bleeding, consider B-Lynch suture, bilateral internal iliac artery ligation and a hysterectomy sooner rather than later (3)

- If facilities are available consider uterine artery embolisation (1)

- Postoperatively, nurse in ICU, repeat FBC, clotting screen, and give thromboprophylaxis (2)

84. A patient is found to be 8 weeks pregnant and has a coil in situ. How would you manage her?

- Give pelvic USS to check fetal viability, site of pregnancy in the uterus or tube, check dates and locate the coil **(3)**

- The coil could have been expelled **(2)**

- If an ectopic pregnancy is suspected, laparoscopy would be diagnostic **(1)**

- If the coil is in the uterine cavity with an intrauterine pregnancy, there is a small risk of infection, miscarriage, ruptured membranes and prematurity **(2)**

- Perform a speculum examination and remove coil if threads are still visible **(2)**

- Warn the patient that there is also a small chance that removal may cause a miscarriage **(2)**

- Conservative management is another option if the strings are not visible and there is a good chance of a successful pregnancy and the coil can be left in **(3)**

- After delivery, arrange for a pelvic radiograph to locate the coil **(2)**

- If it is in the abdomen, arrange for laparoscopic retrieval to prevent adhesion formation **(1)**

- Offer other forms of contraception **(2)**

85. A patient had a caesarean section 6 days ago and comes in with an intensely painful wound and discharging pus from the wound. Describe your management plan.

- Consider the possibility of necrotising fasciitis in an intensely painful wound   (2)

- Take a history to check vomiting and headaches   (2)

- On general examination, check pulse, temperature, BP, and look at the wound for pus, swelling, necrotic tissue, gas gangrene and mark the extent of the erythema with a pen   (3)

- Perform speculum examination and assess lochia for smell; take swabs for microscopy, culture and sensitivity   (2)

- Peform a pelvic USS to detect adnexal masses and collections in the POD   (1)

- Take blood cultures, FBC, CRP, LFTs, U&Es, MSU and wound swabs   (2)

- Start iv fluids, iv antibiotic cover, eg a penicillin or 3rd generation cephalosporin/aminoglycoside/metronidazole combination, and analgesia   (2)

- Remove sutures and promote drainage of pus, applying local antibacterial dressings   (1)

- If necrotising fasciitis or necrotic tissue suspected, arrange for debridement in theatre to remove the dead tissue   (2)

- Chase bacteriology reports and consult microbiologists   (2)

- Consider barrier nursing if she is not responding to antibiotics or risk of MRSA   (1)

- If very ill, the patient may need intensive care as there is a risk of maternal mortality   (1)

86. A 32-year-old nulliparous obese patient had an endometrial biopsy for persistent heavy periods and has been found to have endometrial hyperplasia. Describe your management options.

- Endometrial hyperplasia, especially atypical type, has a high chance of endometrial cancer **(1)**

- Review histology, noting type of hyperplasia if simple, complex, adenomatous or atypical **(2)**

- Note any family history of uterine, breast, ovarian cancer or a history of polycystic ovaries, menstrual history and contraception use **(3)**

- If fertility is desired, give conservative management with high dose Depo-provera 10–20 mg/day for 14 days per month, and repeat endometrial biopsy in 4 months; if hyperplasia still persists, increase dose to 40–80 mg/day and repeat biopsy in 4 months. Depo-provera may cause more weight gain **(4)**

- Alternatively, use Mirena coil which can be left for 5 years and hysteroscopic biopsies are possible while *in situ* **(2)**

- Encourage to lose weight and refer to a dietician **(2)**

- If it persists, take into account history, fertility desire and type of hyperplasia; if atypical offer a hysterectomy **(2)**

- If biopsy normal, continue Depo-provera for 6–12 months and take annual biopsies **(2)**

- If fertility is desired, book for ovulation induction and continue follow-up after delivery **(1)**

- Offer a hysterectomy once family is complete **(1)**

87. **Outline appropriate preoperative work-up for a pelvic mass where malignancy is suspected.**

- Clinical assessment and investigations ensure patient preparation for surgery is optimal **(2)**

- Give counselling and get informed consent **(1)**

- Investigations such as USS, MRI and a CT of abdomen, pelvis and thorax help locate and size tumour, and invasion of other structures **(2)**

- An IVU outlines renal tracts and can reveal obstructive uropathies, and help in staging cervical cancer **(2)**

- A CXR checks for pulmonary metastasis **(2)**

- Tumour markers in ovarian cancer include Ca125 and CEA **(2)**

- A full blood count checks anaemia so it can be corrected before surgery and an X-match of 4 units is appropriate **(2)**

- Obtain liver function tests, urea and electrolytes; check liver and renal status **(2)**

- A clotting screen rules out any coagulation problems **(1)**

- An ECG is needed to check the cardiac status **(1)**

- Respiratory function tests check the lungs for anaesthetic considerations **(1)**

- Get anaesthetic and stoma therapist review **(1)**

- Involve other specialists where other organ systems are involved **(1)**

88. Just before having an emergency caesarean section for fetal distress, the patient requests to be sterilised. She is 28 years old and has four children. How do you manage her request?

- Sterilisation is considered an irreversible procedure **(2)**

- It is recommended that requests for sterilisation should be made at least 1 week before the procedure in the antenatal period with adequate counselling and documentation in the notes **(3)**

- Sterilisation at LSCS is associated with higher regret levels and failure rates than interval sterilisation **(2)**

- Inform the patient that her request may be reasonable but sterilisation needs to be done as an interval procedure in 6 weeks owing to the above reasons **(3)**

- Discuss alternatives and offer Depo-provera injection after delivery **(2)**

- Give leaflets for Mirena coil as coil is as effective as being sterilised; it is effective for 5 years and is reversible **(3)**

- Mention vasectomy, the COCP, the mini-pill as well as implants **(3)**

- Document the discussion in the case notes **(2)**

89. A 34-weeks pregnant woman with two previous caesarean sections requests a vaginal birth. Outline your care plan.

- A previous uterine scar is a risk for uterine rupture during pregnancy and labour **(1)**

- Find out the reasons for the operations and the reason for the request **(1)**

- The risk of uterine rupture with one previous scar is just below 1: 200–300; for two operations the risk is 3% **(2)**

- Inform her that it is not the normal practice in the UK to allow women with two previous LSCSs to deliver vaginally **(2)**

- If she insists, offer a second consultant opinion **(1)**

- If she still wishes vaginal birth, review her regularly and build up her haemoglobin **(2)**

- Record the decision in the notes and that the woman understands the risks involved and that a ruptured uterus may be fatal for mother and baby **(2)**

- IOL with PGs should be avoided as it increases the risk of rupture further **(2)**

- In labour, inform the on-call consultant; do continuous electronic fetal monitoring; offer an epidural; have two large iv access lines; send bloods for FBC and X-match 2 units **(2)**

- Oxytocin augmentation should be avoided; recourse to an early abdominal delivery if labour is dysfunctional **(2)**

- Watch out for signs of uterine rupture; abnormal CTG, maternal tachycardia, cessation of contractions and vaginal bleeding **(2)**

- After delivery, offer contraception including sterilisation **(1)**

90. **What is the psychosexual impact of malignancy on women's health?**

- The diagnosis of malignancy is devastating **(2)**

- The physical state of the disease can cause sexual dysfunction with pain, bleeding, discharge and discomfort affecting intercourse **(2)**

- If there are different forms of therapy eg surgery or radiotherapy, sexual aspects need to form part of the discussion **(2)**

- Radical surgery can lead to psychosexual morbidity with disfigurement, shortening of organs and removal of sex organs **(2)**

- Different forms of treatment can induce a menopausal state **(2)**

- Radiotherapy causes vaginal stenosis and premature menopause, which impacts adversely on women's health **(2)**

- Chemotherapy causes nausea, vomiting, hair loss and reduced libido **(2)**

- Psychiatric morbidity can include depression and anxiety **(2)**

- Adequate counselling at the time of diagnosis and during treatment involving sex therapists is needed **(2)**

- Antidepressants may be needed **(2)**

91. Which patients need a referral to a geneticist?

- Genetic disorders can give congenital malformations, mental retardation, blindness and deafness (3)

- A geneticist can investigate by chromosomal studies and pedigree analysis, risk assess and give counselling (3)

- Ideally prepregnancy counselling is recommended (1)

- Refer couples with a family history or a previous child affected by a genetic or a congenital abnormality (2)

- Conditions that are dominant have a 50% chance of a child being affected, recessive ones 25%, X-linked 25% (males) (3)

- Other conditions to refer are abnormalities on antenatal USS (1)

- Also refer pubertal failure, infertility patients and recurrent miscarriages (2)

- Also refer patients with family history of ovarian, breast, uterine and colonic cancer in 1st degree relatives <50 years old (3)

- Newborns with ambiguous genitalia and dimorphic children need referral (2)

92. **What are the postnatal problems that have significant maternal morbidity and mortality?**

- Maternal morbidity and mortality commonly occur in the puerperium   **(2)**

- VTE remains the major killer of women in the UK in successive enquiries into maternal deaths. Risk assessment is vital and thromboprophylaxis given until women are fully mobile, or for 6 weeks postnatally in those with previous episodes of VTE   **(4)**

- Hypertensive disorders can worsen in the postnatal period, hence observe for 48 hours. Pre-eclampsia/eclampsia and its complications can result in maternal morbidity and mortality, hence prophylactic use of magnesium sulphate is indicated   **(3)**

- Puerperal sepsis is returning, so women with signs of infections should have a complete examination, investigation and antibiotic treatment. The use of prophylactic antibiotics for all caesarean sections is recommended   **(3)**

- Anaemia can cause postpartum collapse, so women who have bled more than normal should have a haemoglobin check before discharge   **(3)**

- Severe postnatal depression can result in suicide, so those women showing signs of severe depression should be seen by a psychiatrist and commenced on treatment. Antenatal recognition of risk factors leads to early detection, referral and treatment   **(3)**

- Postnatal observation can avoid maternal mortality   **(2)**

93. Outline the immediate postoperative complications following gynaecological surgery.

- Careful preoperative assessment can reduce some complications   (2)

- Delayed recovery from anaesthesia with low oxygen saturation   (2)

- Nausea and vomiting – may be drug related   (2)

- Pain and restlessness, raised BP and tachycardia   (3)

- Transfusion reactions with pyrexia and rigors   (3)

- Hypotension from hypovolaemia (bleeding) and cardiac arrhythmias   (2)

- Bowel perforation, pain, peritonitis and abdominal distension   (3)

- Urinary retention, oliguria and ureteric injury with unilateral loin pain and fever   (2)

- Damage to urinary tract may lead to urinary peritonitis   (1)

94. **A 58-year-old woman has a borderline abnormal cervical smear. Describe her management.**

- Cervical screening reduces the incidence and mortality from cervical cancer **(2)**
- Postmenopausal smears can be difficult to obtain and interpret **(2)**
- Take a full history, checking previous cervical abnormalities and abnormal bleeding episodes **(2)**
- Examine the patient and look at the cervix and perform a bimanual examination **(1)**
- Repeat the smear in 6 months **(1)**
- If there are atrophic changes making smear taking difficult, give local oestrogen for 2 weeks then repeat the test **(3)**
- Repeat test in 6 months; if the smear is normal, repeat again in another 6 months and, if normal again, return to normal recall **(2)**
- If still abnormal, refer for colposcopy and biopsy **(2)**
- Offer treatment with large loop excision of the transformation zone and follow up **(2)**
- If diagnostic difficulty, consider a hysterectomy in view of difficulty in obtaining and interpreting cervical smears in postmenopausal women **(3)**

95. **What colposcopic features are used to diagnose cervical intraepithelial neoplasia?**

- A colposcope is a binocular magnifying instrument   (1)

- It allows visualisation of the cervix and squamocolumnar junction   (2)

- Intense and rapid onset of acetowhiting is associated with worsening CIN and HPV infection   (3)

- Large lesions with well-demarcated edges are likely to be high grade CIN   (2)

- Coarse punctation is associated with high-grade CIN   (2)

- High-grade CIN is linked to mosaic lesions   (2)

- Wider intercapillary distance may mean high grade CIN   (2)

- Non-iodine staining areas are likely to be CIN   (3)

- Malignancy is associated with atypical vessels   (3)

96. **Discuss surgical treatment of urodynamic stress incontinence.**

- Any patient having surgery must have urodynamic studies before the procedure, as the surgery may worsen or unmask bladder over activity **(1)**

- Surgical treatment should be offered to those with urodynamic stress incontinence who have had failed conservative management and whose social lives are affected **(3)**

- Burch colposuspension is a most effective surgical operation, with a good success rate of 80–90% at 1 year, but risks include voiding difficulties and overactive bladder. It is a major operation with risks of bleeding, visceral damage, infections and DVT **(3)**

- Sling operations such as TVT and TOT have success rates of 80% at 1 year; they are less invasive than Burch colposuspension, but risks include bladder perforation and voiding problems **(3)**

- Injectable agents are done as a local procedure but have poor success rates of 48% at 1 year **(3)**

- Anterior repair is less successful as an operation for incontinence but is useful if there is prolapse; it is a vaginal procedure **(2)**

- Marshall–Marchetti–Krantz has an unclear role as it is complicated by osteitis pubis **(2)**

- Surgical operations are complicated by voiding difficulties and overactive bladder **(2)**

- Repeat operations may be needed **(1)**

97. **Compare and contrast amniocentesis and chorionic villus sampling.**

- Both are invasive diagnostic tests for fetal karyotyping   **(2)**
- They are done under direct USS guidance   **(1)**
- CVS is performed after 11 weeks with a risk of miscarriage of 2%   **(2)**
- CVS is usually done for maternal age or previous affected child or possible first trimester screening   **(2)**
- Amniocentesis is performed after 16 weeks with a miscarriage risk of 1%   **(2)**
- Amniocentesis usually follows serum screening for high-risk results   **(2)**
- CVS is done in a tertiary centre but an amniocentesis can be done at local level   **(2)**
- Both to be done by a competent person performing the tests frequently   **(1)**
- In multiple pregnancies, both to be done by a specialist in fetomaternal medicine   **(1)**
- CVS is associated with limb hypoplasia and amniocentesis with talipes   **(3)**
- Results in 48 hours for CVS, 2–3 weeks for amniocentesis, but results with FISH or PCR in 48 hours   **(2)**

98. Discuss peritoneal closure after an open abdominal operation.

- Peritoneal healing is complete in 5–6 days   **(2)**
- Peritoneum heals from multiple sites not by apposition of surfaces   **(2)**
- Non-closure of peritoneum shortens operating time   **(2)**
- Earlier return home with non-closure   **(2)**
- Lower rates of postoperative infective morbidity with non-closure   **(2)**
- Less use of analgesia postoperatively with non-closure   **(2)**
- Non-closure leads to quicker return of bowel activity   **(2)**
- Closure increases incidence of adhesions with risk of future problems of bowel obstruction, chronic pain, repeated admissions and difficult operations   **(2)**
- Sutures initiate a foreign body reaction and necroses the peritoneum   **(1)**
- Closure lengthens anaesthesia exposure   **(1)**
- Therefore peritoneal closure is not recommended, as it is associated
  with more risks than benefits   **(2)**

99. **What steps can be taken to resuscitate the distressed fetus in labour?**

- Fetal resuscitation in labour can reduce perinatal morbidity and mortality (2)

- Reduce aortocaval compression by having patient lie on left side, which improves uterine blood flow (3)

- Give oxygen by face mask (1)

- Give intravenous infusion if epidural provoked hypotension (1)

- Stop oxytocin infusion if hyperstimulation occurs or if there is fetal distress (3)

- Tocolysis with terbutaline 0.25 mg sc reverses uterine hyperstimulation (2)

- Alternatively use GTN 0.3–1 mg sublingually (2)

- Amniotic infusion is used to prevent or relieve umbilical cord compression in labour (3)

- Give prompt delivery by a LSCS if a quick vaginal delivery is not possible (3)

100. What are the possible causes of vulval ulcers. How would you manage them?

- Vulval ulcers can be a symptom of serious disease like cancer **(2)**

- Other causes include infections, allergic reactions, systemic disorders and autoimmunity **(3)**

- Take a history to include age, medications, medical conditions, sexual activity, vulval soreness and pain **(3)**

- Clinically examine the ulcer looking at site, size, distribution, discharge, abnormal features and inguinal lymphadenopathy **(4)**

- Investigations to include genital swabs, autoantibodies; if there are suspicious areas then do a vulval biopsy under LA or GA **(3)**

- Treatment should include good hygienic measures and avoidance of synthetic underwear **(1)**

- Give antibiotics, antivirals and antifungals for infections and other treatments depending on the cause **(1)**

- If vulval cancer discovered, refer to oncologists **(2)**

- Referral to dermatologists may be necessary **(1)**

Bibliography

- Cochrane Library *www.cochrane.org*

- Edmonds D. K., *Dewhurst's textbook of obstetrics and gynaecology for postgraduates*, 6th Edn, Oxford: Blackwell Science, 1999.

- Hannah M. E., Hannah W. J., Hewson S. A., Hodnett E. D., Saigal S., Willin A. R. for the Term Breech Trial Collaborative Group 2000. Planned Caesarean section versus planned vaginal birth for breech presentation at term: a randomised multicoated trial. *Lancet* **356**: 1375–83.

- Leusley D. M., Baker P.N., *Obstetrics and gynaecology. An evidence-based text for the MRCOG.* London: Arnold, 2004.

- Nelson-Piercy C. *Handbook of obstetric medicine.* Oxford: ISIS Medical Media, 2000.

- *The Obstetrician & Gynaecologist* (RCOG Press), 2001–2006 (*www.rcog.org.uk/togonline*).

- Royal College of Obstetricians & Gynaecologists. *The Green Top Guidelines*, RCOG Press *www.rcog.org.uk*

- Shafi M., Luesley D., Jordan J. *Handbook of gynaecological oncology.* London: Churchill Livingstone, 2000.

- Sturdee D. *The yearbook of obstetrics & gynaecology, Volume 10.* London: RCOG Press, 2002.

Index

Locators in **bold** type refer to the Questions section, locators in normal type refer to the Answers section.

© 2006 PASTEST

Egerton Court
Parkgate Estate
Knutsford
Cheshire
WA16 8DX

First edition 2006

ISBN 190462796X

ISBN 9781904627968

A catalogue record for this book is available from the British Library.

PasTest Revision Books and Intensive Courses

PasTest has been established in the field of postgraduate medical education since 1972, providing revision books and intensive study courses for doctors preparing for their professional examinations.

Books and courses are available for the following specialties:

MRCGP, MRCP Parts 1 and 2, MRCPCH Parts 1 and 2, MRCPsych, MRCS, MRCOG Parts 1 and 2, DRCOG, DCH, FRCA, PLAB Parts 1 and 2, Dental Students, Dentists and Dental Nurses.

For further details contact:

PasTest, Freepost, Knutsford, Cheshire WA16 7BR

Tel: 01565 752000   **Fax: 01565 650264**

www.pastest.co.uk   **enquires@pastest.co.uk**

Text prepared by Carnegie Book Production Ltd, Lancaster

Printed in the UK by MPG Books Ltd, Bodmin, Cornwall

Concise Practice Essays
for MRCOG 2

Author:
Dr Solwayo Ngwenya MBChB, DFFP, MRCOG
Specialist Registrar in Obstetrics and Gynaecology
Bradford Royal Infirmary
Bradford, UK

Editor:
Mr Stephen Lindow MD, FCOG(SA), FRCOG
Senior Lecturer in Perinatology
Hull University
Consultant Obstetrician and Gynaecologist
Hull Royal Infirmary
Hull, UK

PasTest

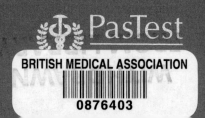